FIRST DO NO HARM

FIRST DO NO HARM

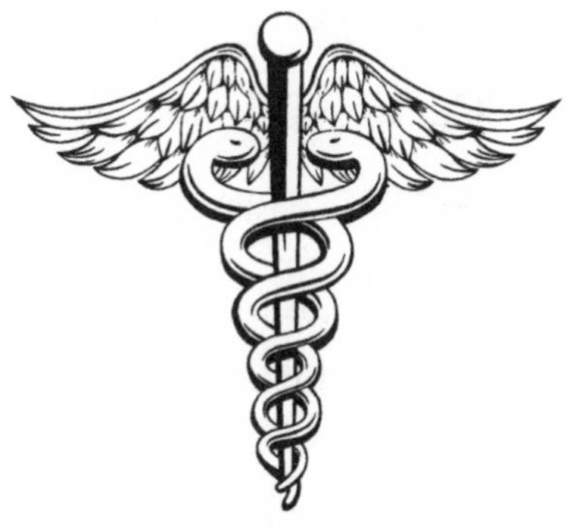

PARACELSUS

Published by

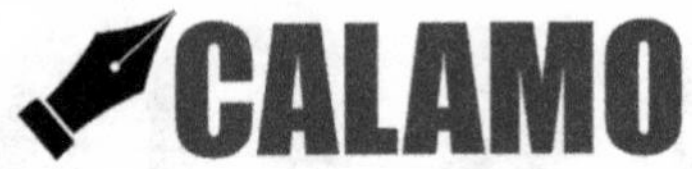

The Calamo Press

Washington D.C.

calamopress.com

Currente-Calamo LLC

2425 17th St NW, Washington D.C. 20009

ISBN 978-1-7351928-7-1

The views and opinions expressed in this book are the author's alone, and do not represent the opinions of any employer, institution, or agency. The content and facts represented herein are accurate as of the time of writing; given that advances in medical knowledge are continuous (particularly with regards to COVID-19), facts, official institutional positions, and other situations may have evolved since then. Therefore, the publisher and the author assume no responsibility for errors, inaccuracies, omissions, or any other inconsistencies herein.

The medical content of this book is for informational purposes only and is not intended to diagnose, treat, cure, or prevent any condition or disease. The stories contained within the book are based on real events but all names, characters, businesses, places, events and incidents have been changed to protect their privacy. Any resemblance to actual persons, living or dead, or actual events is purely coincidental.

TABLE OF CONTENTS

PROLOGUE

The Doctor Will See You Now

Eric begrudgingly took a day off work for the annual doctor visit mandated by his employer-sponsored healthcare insurance. He was an hourly employee but fortunately still had health insurance in his benefits package. However, his co-pay would rise dramatically if he didn't go to this appointment. Still, it seemed unnecessary. He was 45 years old, worked a physical job, didn't smoke, drank socially, and overall felt like he was in great health.

He got up early to go to a commercial lab company for a fasted blood draw the doctor had ordered. *En route* from the lab to the doctor's office he grabbed a coffee and a "breakfast bar" to satisfy his hunger. His wife had been telling him those breakfast bars were low in saturated fat and therefore better than the eggs he really liked.

In the waiting room at the doctor's office, he stared at the diploma and certificates on the wall. MD from Metropolitan University College of Medicine – Eric wondered where that was. Probably some big city in the northeast. There were two framed certificates on the wall, but he couldn't read the font to decipher what they were for. Whatever, he thought, a doctor's a doctor, right?

Once he was back in an exam room and the doctor finally came in, she barely looked at him. She spent most of the time typing on the computer while glancing up briefly to ask him questions.

"You told the nurse your dad had a stroke?"

"Yes, he was a trucker, had a hard life, died in his 50s."

She furrowed her brow as she stared at the computer screen.

The doctor barely examined him – just a quick listen to his heart and lungs, a look at his teeth, eyes, and ears, and some pushes on his belly which aggravated the acid reflux from the coffee and breakfast bar.

"Well, overall I'd say you're doing okay."

Okay? Eric was worried by the tone in her voice.

"In a few years you'll need your first colonoscopy and PSA test, but the only thing right now we need to do is get your cholesterol under control."

"My cholesterol is high?"

"Yes, I'm afraid to say that your LDL is 90, which is above the recommended level of 70. Your total cholesterol is 190, which is right at the upper limit. Given your father's stroke at an early age, and that you already seem to have a good diet low in saturated fat and do physical work for a living, the next step in the medical guidelines is to start you on a statin so you don't have a heart attack or a stroke."

Eric thought of how awful it was for his mom after his dad suddenly died. He didn't want to leave his wife that way.

"Ok."

Eric went straight to the pharmacy to fill the prescription. The pharmacist told him it was for a more expensive brand name statin, but that he should take it instead of the generic because it was more effective and had fewer side effects.

Eric's wife doubled down on decreasing saturated fats in their diet. She loved Eric so much she researched dietary guidelines on the internet. As a result, she started using vegetable oil when cooking dinner, and put low-fat, low-sodium deli meats in the sandwiches she packed him for lunch.

Eric felt weaker at work after starting the statin. He was a packer at a warehouse for a big online retailer, and it was a non-stop physical job. He was able to push through the 12-hour shifts at work, but at home his acid reflux was getting worse and worse.

One night he woke up with a searing pain in his chest. Eric felt like it was difficult to breath. Was this all reflux, or was something wrong? Did he start lowering his cholesterol too late and was this a heart attack?

The pain didn't go away after taking an antacid, and so Eric's wife drove him to the ER, travelling an extra 10 minutes to go to a hospital that advertised it was a center for heart attacks.

Inside the ER, all Eric could think about was his dad. Is this the kind of place his dad died in? The triage nurse immediately did an EKG, put an IV in his arm and drew labs, and then led him and his wife to the waiting room, where they would spend the next 4 hours.

Finally, at 6 am he was brought back into the real ER where he was given a private room. The ER doctor who came to see him was a jolly older man, who spent time examining Eric and talking to him and his wife.

"I really think you just have terrible acid reflux. We're going to give you a GI cocktail and repeat an EKG in 2 hours and make sure this isn't an evolving atypical heart attack. I do want to let you know that we change shifts at 7 AM, so you'll probably be seeing a colleague of mine at 8 AM after that repeat EKG."

Eric felt reassured by this doctor.

At 8 AM a tech came in to repeat his EKG, then whisked off to give it to the morning ER doctor. When that ER doctor opened Eric's electronic medical record in the computer a bright warning appeared.

CHEST PAIN ALERT!

PATIENT HAS NOT HAD CHEST X-RAY

-> *Order Chest X-Ray*

PATIENT HAS NOT HAD REPEAT TROPONIN -> *Order Troponin*

DOES PATIENT NEED CARDIOLOGY CONSULT? -> *Consult Cardiology*

"These God damn alerts" he muttered. He clicked on orders for a Chest X-Ray and a repeat troponin (a test that is elevated in heart attacks), as well as liver enzymes, which came back elevated.

The morning doctor went to see him Eric for the first time. Eric's chest pain was the same – he kept feeling a heavy weight in his chest. But Eric wasn't sure, maybe it was anxiety, the growing fear that he would end up like his father.

"Given that your pain is no better, I think we should admit you for observation. We can have a cardiologist come by to see you as well."

Eric was admitted to the hospital and later that morning the cardiology team came to see him. It was an impressive looking group, with an attending physician, a nurse practitioner, a resident doctor, and a medical student. The attending cardiologist talked so fast that Eric could barely understand him. It didn't help that the cardiologist directed most of the conversation towards Eric's wife, who was exhausted.

"Given your history, and that the statins aren't making you any better, the most definitive thing we can offer is a cardiac catheterization. It's a minimally invasive procedure, where we thread a little wire up a blood vessel in your groin and make

double sure there are no blockages in your heart. This is really the only way to know whether or not this chest pain is from the heart."

Seeing that his wife was getting scared, Eric interjected, "*What are the risks of the procedure?*"

"Ah, good question! There is always the risk of bleeding from the blood vessel in the groin, and infection, which are minimal. We do several of these procedures every day and we are accredited as a regional cardiac catheterization center."

That sounded legitimate.

"And, of course, you are given some sedation and pain medications, and so there is always the risk of a reaction to the medications, but it'll be an anesthesiologist who manages all that."

Sleep-deprived and anxious, Eric agreed to the cardiac catheterization.

Eric remembered the anesthesiologist telling him he would sleep well as he got the sedation medication in the pre-op room. The next thing he remembered was a frantic voice yelling, *"WAKE UP! BREATHE! BREATHE!"*

The catheterization had gone off without a hitch. But apparently when Eric awoke after the procedure, he had mumbled something about being in pain. A brand-new nurse called the resident doctor on the cardiology team, who ordered 2 mg of hydromorphone, a powerful opioid. Eric had never taken an opioid before in his life, and right after the nurse pushed the hydromorphone into his IV, he stopped breathing.

The nurse freaked out and called a Code Blue, and in moments a bevy of doctors came flying into the surgery recovery unit. One of them gave Eric the opioid reversal drug naloxone, and soon Eric began to breathe again. All the while, Eric's wife had no idea what was going on.

The cardiac catheterization showed no blockages and a totally healthy heart.

Months later, Eric and his wife had put the hospital stay behind them. He was still taking his statin and was due soon for repeat labs to check his liver enzymes.

Then a thick envelope arrived in the mail: The hospital bill.

It took Eric and his wife a good 30 minutes to sift through all the pages and figure out what insurance had paid for, and what charges would be billed to Eric. Of the ones billed to Eric, there were two concerning items:

$2,000 for Critical Care, Procedure Code 99291

and

$5,000 for Magill Anesthesia Associates services

Eric and his wife stared at the bill with dread. He had missed so much work because of the hospital stay that other bills were piling up. Eric didn't have any time off during business hours, so it was his wife who called the toll-free number listed on the bill.

The Critical Care charge was for the Code Blue team who brought Eric back to life with Narcan. Eric's wife pointed out that it was the hospital (really the resident doctor, and the nurse who failed to question the dose) who had overdosed him on an opioid, so none of that was Eric's fault. The insurance customer service rep didn't seem surprised by the story and said she would file a claim with the hospital disputing the charge.

The $5,000 charge for Magill Anesthesia Associates was more problematic. It turns out that while the hospital Eric went to was in-network for his insurance plan, the anesthesiology team were outside contractors hired by the hospital and out-of-network. Magill Anesthesia Associates' services were NOT covered by Eric's insurance.

Eric's wife was livid. No one had told them this. In fact, Eric barely talked to the anesthesiologist, he'd just swooped in right before the cardiac catheterization, gotten consent for anesthesia, and then put Eric to sleep. The insurance rep was quick to point out the various payment plans they offered for situations like this. Eric's wife was distraught but took notes on the payment plans and their interest rates, which varied from 5 - 20%.

Payment plan selected, once again Eric and his wife tried to put the whole thing behind him. He was having trouble paying off the anesthesia bill and had become cynical about the benefits of healthcare insurance. Still, Eric was glad it was over and grateful it had happened in 2019, before the COVID-19 chaos of 2020.

All the while, Eric dutifully continued to take the statin.

As the waves of COVID-19 ebbed and flowed, Eric found himself overdue for his annual physical for work. For all his new doubts about the healthcare system, the prospect of paying more for insurance or losing his employer-sponsored plan was scarier still, and he arranged for a quick telemedicine visit with his doctor. She ordered labs to check his liver enzymes and cholesterol and scheduled him for a proper office visit to examine him and discuss the results.

Back at her office, Eric felt an uncomfortable sense of déjà vu.

"Your liver enzymes are still elevated but stable – that is a known side effect of statins. But your cholesterol is coming down, so if that continues to drop, we can think about weaning you off the statin."

Finally, some good news, thought Eric.

"I see here you are due for your annual flu shot, as well as your first COVID-19 vaccine. We can get both of those taken care of right now."

Eric was pretty sure he'd had COVID-19 over the summer, when the virus had run rampant through the warehouse where he worked. He had felt very tired one day and lost his sense of taste and smell that week.

"I already had COVID. I think I'm good."

"I'm sorry to hear that. But what we know from studies and guidance from the NIH, CDC, and FDA, is that while you may have some natural immunity against COVID, the vaccines will provide you with additional protection, and decrease your chances of getting COVID."

"I don't understand, I had COVID already, I'm immune."

"You don't want to get it again and give it to someone you love who dies, do you?"

Eric looked at the doctor, realizing she had set him on a path that resulted in a needless invasive procedure, a brush with death, and bills that were about to go to a collections agency. Yet his troubles were nothing to her – she had no connection with him, he was just the "10:30 AM appointment."

"I'm good, thanks."

And with that, Eric stood up and walked out, never to return.

INTRODUCTION

"Modern medicine is a negation of health. It isn't organized to serve human health, but only itself, as an institution. It makes more people sick than it heals."

—Ivan Illich

"County ER? This is Rescue 4. We are incoming from a nursing home with a 76-year-old male. He's a COVID alert AND a stroke alert. He has baseline dementia so staff unable to say how altered he is, but last seen normal two days ago. Also has cough, fever, and shortness of breath. Oxygen is 92% on 4 liters nasal cannula. We'll be at your back door in 5 minutes, over."

Early reports from China on the clinical manifestations of COVID-19 focused on lung disease. However, for clinicians like myself, it became apparent early in the pandemic that there were also blood clots and neurologic issues in severe COVID-19 infections. Many scientists now believe that COVID-19 primarily damages blood vessels, causing dysfunction in the lungs, heart, brain, and other organs. That explains why this nursing home resident coming to the ER was experiencing altered mental status and difficulty breathing.

I remember this patient very well. When EMS brought him into the ER, he was breathing heavily and looked sleepy at the same time. His oxygen levels bounced around from 89-95%, so we kept him on supplemental oxygen through a nasal cannula, rather than escalate respiratory support. Fortunately for the patient it was mid-2020, and early intubation had fallen out of favor, at least in my hospital. It was still early enough in the pandemic, however, that I had to argue with the radiology technicians about doing a computed tomography (CT) scan of his head to evaluate what was causing his altered mental status. Until the Delta wave in 2021, many hospital personnel were quite choosy about whether they would come into contact with a COVID-19 patient. In the ER, of course, we had no such luxury of choice. I told the CT techs they could leave the room while we put the patient in the scanner and figured out what buttons to push ourselves. They relented.

In the ER we joke about CT scans emitting "therapeutic radiation," and this patient did become more awake after the CT. There was no brain bleed on the images, so I went off to make a host of phone calls to neurology, the hospitalist, and the patient's family to inquire about his baseline mental status and update them on a likely hospital admission. Meanwhile, in and out of the patient's dark, closed-door room, masked, gowned, and gloved nurses went about drawing blood and tinkering with his oxygen support. As the patient became more and more alert, to him it perhaps seemed like evil scientists from a horror film were poking and prodding him.

Making matters worse was the TV in his room, which was set on our default hospital channel, with creepy and tone-deaf videos of the hospital CEO talking about lockdowns, social distancing, and hospital visitor restrictions. The patient in his COVID-19 and dementia-induced haze looked around an unfamiliar and bizarre environment and must've thought he'd been kidnapped by aliens.

"Sir! Sir! STOP! Get back in your room! You have COVID!"

When the charge nurse started yelling, I looked up from my computer to see the man standing outside his room in the ER hallway. He was barefoot and his hospital gown was open in the back. His IV was dripping blood and the nasal cannula tubing had been ripped away from the oxygen port in the wall and was twisted around his neck. He looked scared, darting his eyes around wildly. It was mere seconds before he tore off his hospital gown and took off running completely naked down the ER hallway.

"Go stop him! Call security!"

Charge nurses, the medical "Karens", live for moments like this.

To the patient's credit, he made it as far as the ER waiting room where the security guard posted at the entrance quickly stopped him and escorted him back into the ER. The patient's naked, COVID-19-positive appearance in the waiting room caused more than a few people to reassess their emergent need for medical care and leave. And the patient's sprint down the hall confirmed for me that his oxygen needs were minimal.

The patient calmed down and was admitted. He required supplemental oxygen for 5 days. He stayed in the hospital for 4 weeks, however, because he couldn't go back to the nursing home until he had two negative COVID-19 polymerase chain reaction (PCR) tests 48 hours apart, and there was simply nowhere else for him to go.

That patient's instinct to literally run away from our medical system was correct. We in the ER had become so accustomed to our dystopian doctoring in space suits that we failed to anticipate how scary the situation looked to the patient. Beyond terrifying appearances, the odds of medical care doing more harm than good are also frightening. That was true before the COVID-19 pandemic, and very true during it. And unless drastic changes are made, it will also be true into the future.

Indeed, the response to COVID-19 has revealed the depths of mismanagement and dysfunction that pervade the American medical establishment. Government bureaucracies fumbled in their actions while politicizing a microscopic virus. Pharmaceutical and insurance companies greedily took advantage of new demand for their products and services. And while government ineptitude and corporate profiteering are not surprising, the incompetence and hive mentality demonstrated by individual doctors, healthcare organizations, and medical professional societies caught many Americans off-guard.

Despite that, a surprising number of Americans seem ready to dismiss the pandemic's revelations as a one-off phenomenon. Two-thirds of respondents to a 2021 survey said they trusted the United States' (US) healthcare system. Another 2021 poll found that 59% of respondents *gained* confidence in their doctors during the COVID-19 pandemic.

How is that possible? The relationship between doctors and patients seems now to be more abusive than healing. For decades patients dutifully showed up for their annual physical, only to be prescribed harmful drugs like statins. When patients needed honest, trustworthy medical advice during COVID-19, many doctors and medical organizations repeated often-contradictory talking points from cable news anchors and career government bureaucrats.

The truth is doctors today are highly educated but poorly trained. Medical education has devolved from a rigorous and elite process to a fail forward system. Doctors who graduate from that system are not independent thinkers and healers, but rather dutiful foot soldiers who follow their marching orders.

Many of those marching orders come from professional medical societies. These groups were always progressive, but now they no longer need to hide their ideology. *"The sky is lavender!"* those societies proclaim, as their clinical guidelines become increasingly political and less and less scientific.

Meanwhile, healthcare organizations and hospitals are filled with administrators who are living embodiments of the Peter Principle: they have risen to their level of incompetence. Keeping them afloat are unnecessary procedures and financial agreements with insurance companies that ensure corporate health at the expense of patient health.

The government agencies supposedly regulating this system are no different from the rest of the US federal government – in the late stages of decomposition. Thus, the Centers for Disease Control and Prevention (CDC) and the National Institutes of Health (NIH) perpetuate problems to perpetuate their existence. Meanwhile, the Food and Drug Administration (FDA) is caught in regulatory capture by pharmaceutical companies, who always manage to emerge victorious whether or not their products work as advertised.

What is vitally important for the public to realize is that the response to COVID-19 demonstrates how medicine operates every day, not just during a pandemic. The entire healthcare system is one that rewards compliance over competence.

So don't believe the talking heads when they proclaim, "*Without us, it would've been so much worse.*" Before the COVID-19 pandemic, the US healthcare system was suffering from falling standards – COVID-19 merely amplified and publicized pre-existing problems.

I wrote this book for people who are now questioning whether they should trust their individual doctors and our healthcare system. To describe incidents that are hidden from public view, as a medical insider I've also included stories that help paint the entire picture of our healthcare system's dysfunction. Those stories are based on real events, but identifying details have been changed to protect privacy.

Unfortunately, our entire healthcare system is rotten, and that decay now extends to individual doctors who blindly do what they're told instead of thinking critically. For your health and that of your loved ones, it is you who needs to think critically about healthcare.

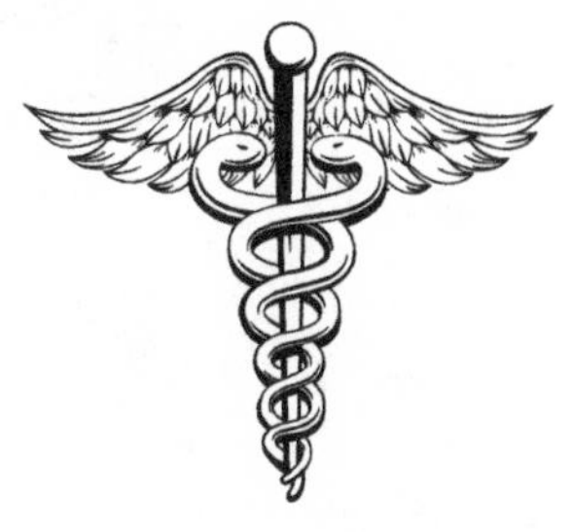

MEDICAL EDUCATION & TRAINING: FAILING FORWARD

"Finish last in your league and they call you idiot. Finish last in medical school and they call you doctor."

—Abe Lemons

Most of the American public admires and has faith in physicians. The popular view of doctors is that they are brilliant, selfless, hard-working individuals who will sacrifice everything to heal their patients. For most patients, the sight of a physician in a white coat, seemingly confident and all-knowing, is reassuring.

And the place where it all begins, medical school, is believed to be the toughest and most rigorous professional school, a seeming guarantee of competence. And even though most people do not understand the particulars of post-medical school residency and fellowship training, the prevailing view is that doctors who have undergone such training can be universally trusted. Therefore, people also believe medical errors by doctors are rare.

I'm not here to bash all doctors (I am one after all), but I am going to break the news that the physician population is more heterogeneous than you may think, and that is because medical education is not what it once was.

Medical education in the US has evolved from informal apprenticeships teaching bloodletting with leeches, to the pioneering Johns Hopkins medical school model that produced the trusted family doctor, to what it is now: a pass-fail system where nearly everyone passes.

Medical education is no longer focused on training physicians to heal a variety of conditions. Superseding medicine is the corporate aim of ensuring a steady supply of cheap hospital labor and the academic aim of accreditation. The current motto for medical education and training is not the Hippocratic oath, but rather, "we fail forward."

When I applied to medical school, I thought it would be the most rigorous academic venture I would undertake. I expected to spend the first two years of medical school inside a classroom, learning the ins and outs of human anatomy and physiology. I expected to spend all of my third and fourth year inside the hospital learning how to be a doctor.

My first hint that something was amiss with what I thought was a selective endeavor came during the application process. When I traveled to medical schools for interviews and made small talk with the other applicants, I became nervous. I had applied to 5 medical schools, but most applicants I talked to had applied to 10, 15, or even 20 schools. Applying to 20 schools seemed excessive – all you need is one acceptance to become a doctor. I shrugged that off with my first acceptance letter and headed to medical school excited and nervous about all the hard work that was yet to come.

The reality of medical school proved to be quite different. Although I spent some time in anatomy lab dissecting cadavers, I spent most of the first two years of medical school on the couch watching lectures online. It turns out the students ahead of me had complained about not having lectures recorded and that the temperature in the medical school auditorium was frigid. The school administrators folded instantly, making classroom attendance optional and recording all lectures so they could be viewed online.

I always thought it odd that in response to a few complaints my medical school threw out lecture attendance and made interacting with instructors completely optional for the first two years. It wasn't until later that I realized the school's accreditation depended in part on students' perception of how complaints were handled. It turns out that a medical school's accreditation evaluation includes results from a survey of graduating students. That survey asks questions about how well administrators help students with academic difficulties, how much time medical students have for leisure activities, and even how much the medical students like the student lounge!

As I found out later in my career, bad responses to any of those questions, whether the question was legitimate or ridiculous, spell trouble for a medical school's accreditation prospects.

Therefore, while medical schools hold the keys to the kingdom during the admissions process, once students are granted admission, the power dynamic shifts towards the students. Administrators are heavily incentivized to make sure that all medical students are happy and graduate, regardless of performance. Thus, medical school admission is the tightest funnel in the process to becoming a doctor, and even that funnel is wider than you think.

The longstanding belief that while many people aspire to be a doctor, it is extraordinarily difficult to get into medical school conflicts with the truth. Just how selective is medical school these days? US medical schools accept between 1% - 20% of their applicants, which seems exclusive. Yet those statistics are from the vantage point of the medical school. From the viewpoint of the applicant, the acceptance rate hovers around 40%, and that is just for allopathic medical schools.

It turns out there are two types of US medical schools – allopathic and osteopathic. Many applicants apply to both, and it's likely that more than 40% of applicants gain acceptance to a US medical school. The reason for the gap between school acceptance rates and an individual applicant's chance of admission is that aspiring doctors apply to double digit numbers of medical schools.

However, even if a 40% chance of admission to a stateside medical school is not good enough, there is always the Caribbean. Those who can remember Operation Urgent Fury from the early 1980s may have wondered why the US had to send special forces soldiers to rescue American medical students in Grenada. It turns out that the small Caribbean Island had two main sources of income: cash crops and producing doctors. At the time of the US invasion in 1983, the St. George's University School of Medicine had about 700 American medical students. That generated between 10-15% of Grenada's national GDP.

St. George's University School of Medicine opened its doors in 1976 and was a pioneer in offshore medical education for those who couldn't get into a stateside medical school. There are now dozens of Caribbean medical schools with deceptively American-sounding names like: Georgetown American University in Grenada, Ross University School of Medicine in Barbados, Xavier University School of Medicine in Aruba, and Metropolitan University College of Medicine in Antigua. And despite most of those Caribbean institutions being for-profit, tuition can be still be subsidized with US federal student loans.

Although many Caribbean schools do not publish their admission statistics, the more "prestigious" Caribbean schools claim acceptance rates of 40 - 44%. Again, that acceptance rate is from the view of the school. Thus, an applicant rejected from stateside medical schools could apply to multiple Caribbean medical schools and have a much greater than 40% chance of securing an acceptance.

Why should Americans care about young aspiring doctors going to the Caribbean for their medical education? Objectively, Caribbean medical school graduates have lower board exam pass rates and a harder time matching into residency. Subjectively, in my experience, while there are some great Caribbean-trained doctors, the quality of most reflects why they were rejected from stateside medical schools in the first place.

Yet Caribbean medical students graduate with the coveted MD degree and a diploma without any mark of their sub-par training. That deception continues in perpetuity, as the average patient likely views someone with an allopathic degree (MD) from Ross University as a superior doctor to someone with a stateside osteopathic degree (DO).

Those in favor of offshore medical schools will argue that Caribbean medical students fly to US hospitals for their clinical rotations during the third and fourth years of medical school. Some will argue that Caribbean-educated students still need to match into a US residency program. Others will argue that regardless of where they are trained, medical students still need to graduate medical school. However, whether stateside or beachside, today medical school is a fail forward system with hardly anyone ever flunking out.

And as we shall see, as more subpar applicants are admitted to medical schools, more subpar doctors will graduate to treat patients.

"Do you like to party?"

What an odd question to ask someone at a party.

"Uh, yeah, I'm here right?"

Jane giggled and walked away after my awkward answer. I was at a house party with my medical school classmates. Spending the first two years of medical school on the couch watching lectures online had given us plenty of free time to enjoy ourselves. Nothing wrong with a "work hard, play hard" mentality, though I suspected Jane's question had to do with the drug use that was becoming an issue for her and some other classmates. I saw Jane disappear into the bathroom with a creepy law school student who always showed up at our parties.

During my third year of med school I was paired with a student named Charlie for our surgery rotation. A typical morning involved arriving at 5 am to "pre-round" on patients and help the residents with their notes. Despite the early mornings, Charlie always seemed *very* awake. I relied on espresso to get me through medical school, but no amount of caffeine ever got me as excited as Charlie. Charlie wanted to be a neurosurgeon, so I assumed he was popping ADD meds and "gunning" for good letters of recommendation, since our pass-fail grades made it hard to distinguish oneself for competitive specialties like neurosurgery.

One day Charlie had car trouble and asked if I would give him a ride to and from the hospital. Sure, no problem. I remember that his bag was a mess, overflowing with crumbled papers and loose credit cards. Charlie had a lot of credit cards.

After my surgery rotation was over, I was on an easy elective and tried to get my life in order. I set about cleaning my dirty car. While I was vacuuming underneath the passenger seat, I found a plastic bag containing a white powder. So the rumors were true, Charlie did more than just ADD meds. I was angry – what if by chance I had been pulled over by a cop? I would be in serious trouble while Charlie would still be snorting cocaine on his way to see patients.

Jane and Charlie both had issues throughout medical school with erratic behavior, and they did terrible in our "Doctoring" class where we were observed interacting with real patients. But terrible was still good enough for a passing grade.

Jane wanted to be an ophthalmologist, which like neurosurgery is a very competitive specialty. However, Jane's dreams were dashed and she is now a primary care doctor. Charlie, somehow, is a neurosurgeon.

Imagine you run a medical school. Your stated mission is to educate and train the best new doctors. However, you also need to keep everyone involved in the medical school employed – and that includes those at associated research centers and laboratories that bring in lucrative government grants.

As a seasoned administrator, you are aware that the Liaison Committee on Medical Education (LCME - the main medical school accreditation organization) makes you report student graduation, attrition, and dismissal rates. You know that during each 8-year accreditation cycle you must report every time a student has to repeat a class or do any remediation. You are also deathly afraid of the graduating medical student survey that asks the students how well the school assisted them with any academic difficulties. You have heard horror stories from colleagues about the heavy weight the LCME places on the student survey responses.

Hence, the Catch-22 is that if you as an administrator enforce high standards for medical students, inevitably some students will falter and fail. If you dare to fail a student, the medical school's accreditation will be in peril, jeopardizing the research programs and government grants. Now you understand that the real mission of running a medical school is keeping the lights on. The unspoken incentive of every medical school is for all students to graduate and match into a residency program.

Does that incentive translate into high graduation rates? Yes – 96% of medical students graduate. Is there any concrete evidence of poor medical student performance and how it is handled? Not really. Forget trying to figure out if your surgeon got a 'D' in their surgery rotation - medical school grades have been pass-fail for decades now. That pass-fail system makes it easy for sub-par students to graduate and successfully match into a residency program.

The fail forward model continues after medical school to residency. (Everything said here about residency equally applies to fellowship training, which is sub-specialty training that some doctors do after residency). But before we discuss how residents fail forward in a similar manner to medical students, what is residency and why do new doctors need to do it?

Medical school graduates are doctors in name only. Filled with esoteric book knowledge, new doctors have no clue how to order medications, work with nurses (i.e., listen to nurses), and tease out a diagnosis from a confusing history and equivocal physical exam. In other words, a new doctor on day one of his surgery residency is no more skilled in operating than a toddler playing the game Operation. Hence the purpose of residency: to teach the actual skills of doctoring.

Residency follows an apprenticeship model where residents treat patients under an attending physician's supervision. While medical school is general, residency is specialized (i.e., pediatrics, surgery, neurology, etc.). Soon-to-graduate medical students apply to residency in a chosen specialty through a process called the Match.

The Match reinforces the fail forward process and is very different from a typical school or job application. Although medical students choose what residency programs they apply to, they do not choose what residency program they enter. After the applications and interviews are completed, medical students rank the residency programs they interviewed at, and residency programs rank the medical students they interviewed. The Match then pairs students with residency programs using those rank order lists.

The actual matching is done with a proprietary algorithm run by the National Residency Matching Program (NRMP). NRMP's headquarters is located on K Street in Washington, DC. It's at a site which is surrounded by hospital lobbyists and within walking distance of the American Medical Association's (AMA) Washington office. Therefore, it is not surprising that when entering the Match, medical students must sign a contract binding them to work wherever they are matched and forbidding salary negotiations (essentially signing up for 3 - 6 years of work at less than a minimum wage).

It is hospitals who win several times over with the Match. One, hospitals gain valuable physician labor at a cheap and fixed rate. Two, it is the federal government who actually pays for the majority of residents' salaries through Medicare's Direct Graduate Medical Education program. Three, hospitals with residency programs receive additional Medicare funds through Indirect Medical Education payments. And lastly, the Match fills over 95% of all open hospital residency positions.

The Match is also shockingly efficient at letting poor performing medical students become primary care doctors. To understand how this happens, it is important to know that matching all students into a residency is a key statistic in a medical school's accreditation evaluation. Therefore, before the Match there is a not-so-subtle push by medical school administrators for poor performing medical students to choose residency specialties that are less competitive and easier to match into. That is how my classmate Jane with her dreams of becoming an ophthalmologist ended up as a family medicine doctor.

Why family medicine? The reality is primary care specialties like family medicine, internal medicine, and pediatrics are not competitive because their future salary prospects are lower than competitive specialties like neurosurgery. Reflecting that, it can be tough for hospitals to fill their primary care residency positions. Therefore, medical school and hospital incentives align when it comes to filling primary care spots, especially if it's with subpar medical students.

You may go your entire life without needing a neurosurgeon, but at some point, you will likely receive primary care. Our perverted medical training system fills niche specialties with the best and brightest, while encouraging poor performing students to fail forward into the specialties that see the most patients. The end result for primary care is fewer quality doctors, and another weak link in our collapsing healthcare system.

I was looking forward to a rare Saturday night off work. As a resident, I only got four days off a month, including weekends. I had plans to eat real food, drink a beer, and sleep for 12 hours.

My phone rang. Caller ID said it was our chief resident. The chief resident deals with filling vacancies when someone calls out sick, or as in this case, calls out for other reasons.

"Can you pick up a shift tonight?"

I wanted so badly to get a full night's rest. On the other hand, an extra shift means extra pay, and my student loans with interest compounding had recently topped $200,000.

"Who is it for?"

"For Sarah."

Oh Sarah. She had a track record of mixing up her moonlighting and residency shifts. (Moonlighting is when residents or fellows work shifts at another hospital outside of their primary job duties.) We were allowed to moonlight, but it wasn't supposed to ever interfere with our residency shifts.

"She moonlighting tonight?"

Long pause. Being a chief resident is a stepping-stone for a future hospital administrative position. My question was making the aspiring middle manager uncomfortable. However, Sarah had burned so many bridges over the years that I got the full story.

"No, she's supposed to work here tonight. Last night she went out downtown, got drunk and out of control again. This time the bar called the cops on her and she started mouthing off to the cop. He arrested her so now she's in jail for drunk and disorderly conduct. The program directors are working on bailing her out."

WOW. Everybody knew Sarah liked to have a good time (especially the orthopedic surgery residents). And I knew she was an outspoken Northeastern progressive who hated the cops. But I didn't know our residency program directors would bail someone out of jail. And I couldn't imagine what kind of professional consequences Sarah was about to face.

I worked the shift, made some cash, and then in my chronic sleep-deprived state I forgot about the incident. A few months later I was on a rotation in the ICU with Sarah on my team. One day after a shift she asked if I wanted to go out for drinks. I joked, *"Sure, as long as you behave yourself."* Sarah laughed. After a few drinks I asked if anything had happened after the arrest. Sarah shrugged, *"Charges dropped, program directors said don't do it again."*

That was it?! "Don't do this again?!"

Yes, that was it. Sarah managed to avoid getting arrested for another year, and we both graduated together in the same residency class. As far as residency credentials go, she and I look identical on paper - same training at the same institution.

There is bad news and good news when it comes to residency.

The bad news is that residency does not filter out bad or even dangerous doctors.

The good news is that residency's intense work hours transfer at least some medical knowledge. Because of those long hours, until a few decades ago many residents found it expedient to simply live in the hospital. When I completed residency, most weeks had two or three 30-hour shifts. As scary as it may sound to have a 26-year-old who's been a doctor for six months treating your grandmother's heart failure after being awake for 30 hours, in such an immersive system most residents cannot help but learn at least the basics of their specialty.

However, that old system overworked many residents. And in keeping with the loosening of standards in other fields like the military, the Accreditation Council for Graduate Medical Education (ACGME – the organization that accredits residency programs), is on a mission to make residency more of an experience in health and wellness than a time of intense learning. And in the name of health and wellness (for residents, not for patients), the ACGME now enforces strict resident work hour limitations.

However, the origins of the ACGME's residency work hour restrictions came not from genuine concerns for residents' health, but from a tragic case of medical error that resulted in the death of a young woman.

That case happened in 1984, when a college freshman named Libby Zion was admitted to a New York hospital with a flu-like illness and strange jerking movements. The residents treating her overnight administered an opioid, and then after she became increasingly agitated, administered an antipsychotic. By the next morning Libby had a temperature of 107°F, went into cardiac arrest, and died. It turns out Libby had been taking an antidepressant, which when combined with the opioid and the antipsychotic given by the residents, resulted in serotonin syndrome, a medication reaction that causes agitation, abnormal movements, hyperthermia, and eventually heart arrhythmias and death. Part of the outrage surrounding Libby Zion's death was that the residents who treated Libby were in the middle of a 36-hour shift. In response to a slew of civil and criminal litigation, in 1989 New York State limited work hours for medical residents to no more than 80 hours per week, and no more than 24 hours in a row.

A full thirteen years later, in 2003, the ACGME decided that they too were outraged by the death of Libby Zion, and they adopted those same work hour limitations for all accredited residency programs in the US.

Eighty hours per week is still a lot of work, and there were legitimate safety issues with traditional resident work hours. However, the ACGME's new work hour restrictions may be making patient care more dangerous. The work hour restrictions have resulted in increased patient hand-offs as residents who reach the end of their shifts must transfer patient care over to another resident. If that sounds dangerous, it is. Patient handoffs are a moment when crucial information can be overlooked, and a major risk factor for serious medical errors.

The full consequences of resident work hour restrictions on patient care and the quality of doctors are not yet fully known. The generation of doctors trained since the early 2000s is not yet the majority of today's physician workforce. But eventually all doctors will have been trained in a system that says when the clock strikes midnight, the attitude is "not my patient, not my problem."

Aside from work hour limitations, the ACGME's obsession with promoting wellness and preventing burnout has eradicated any real standards for evaluating residents' performance. While helping young physicians successfully navigate residency is a noble cause, the response of the ACGME (like many other American institutions) is to water down standards.

To follow medical school grades which are pass-fail, the ACGME has devised a resident grading system called the "Milestones." Scaled from 1 to 5, the trademarked Milestones are reminiscent of infant developmental stages (e.g., Level 1 you can roll over, Level 5 you can walk and chew toys at the same time). Except that residents are playing with patients' lives, not toys.

The Milestones could be a functioning grading system if there were some way to differentiate between the levels. However, in reality, all the Milestones vary from "good" to "great" and don't contain any level that describes sub-par performance. Even so, the Milestones system could be functional if there were consequences for not achieving Level 5 status by the end of residency. However, in practice, if a soon-to-graduate resident is at the Level 4 rather than the Level 5 Milestone, that's OK. They will still go on to graduate residency and practice medicine independently.

And just how many residents graduate to become independent doctors? Residency graduation rates are firewalled by the ACGME, but survey data from the AAMC shows that between 71-78% of medical school graduates completed residency within 4 years. Of note, many residencies are 5 or

6 years in length, so that number is a gross underestimation of true residency graduation rates, which again, are obscured by the ACGME. The AAMC also reports that the number of residency programs in the US is increasing, demonstrating the push to graduate more residency-trained physicians (i.e., more cheap hospital labor).

While the medical schools' fail forward system is already concerning, when residents fail forward the stakes are even higher, as doctors who graduate residency go on to practice medicine without any oversight.

"Could you page GI, please?"

I was treating a patient with a bad gastrointestinal (GI) bleed. I had given medications to help stop the bleeding, but what the patient really needed was an endoscopy by a GI doctor.

The phone rang a few minutes later.

"This is Shelly for Dr. Lewis."

I assumed Shelly was the GI doctor's physician assistant (PA).

"Hi Shelly, we've got a GI bleed in room 8. I'm going to need you all to come see her. She was slightly hypotensive at first but responded well to IV fluids."

"Ok, we'll be right down."

Shelly and Dr. Lewis arrived quickly and went to see the patient. Dr. Lewis looked dishevelled in his scrubs, but Shelly looked very professional in her business casual attire.

When they emerged from the patient's room, Dr. Lewis was on the phone arranging for anesthesia and an operating room for the endoscopy. I turned to Shelly.

"What do you think caused it? She has no medical history and she's not an alcoholic, so it's not varices."

(Varices are enlarged veins of the esophagus that form in a variety of conditions, including alcoholic liver disease.)

Shelly looked uncomfortable.

"I'm actually not medical. You should ask Dr. Lewis when he gets off the phone."

I got called into another patient room and didn't get to talk to Dr. Lewis before he left. I later asked one of the nurses who Shelly was.

"You don't know? That's his minder."

"His minder?"

"Yes, he apparently hit on some female patients and a couple times grabbed the scrub tech's ass in the OR. Shelly was assigned by the hospital to follow him around everywhere so he behaves."

"Why isn't he suspended or fired?"

"He makes the hospital too much money."

"You know, she answered his pager when I called."

"That's hilarious. Maybe one day she will become his PA."

Perhaps more troubling than the failure to enforce high standards during medical education and training is the failure of the practicing medical profession to filter out its bad apples. This is truly a shame as it sullies by association the good doctors who are still practicing great medicine. Short of sexual assault, running an opioid pill-mill, or defrauding Medicare for millions of dollars, it's extremely difficult for a doctor to lose their medical license. (Although during the COVID-19 pandemic, many doctors were threatened with losing their license after writing ivermectin prescriptions.) Even medical malpractice lawsuits don't cleanse the profession, as evidenced by reports to the National Practitioner Data Bank (NPDB).

The NPDB is a database of medical malpractice payments and disciplinary actions taken against physicians. It is understandable that during a long career, even a good doctor could get sued once or twice. However, looking at malpractice payments from 1990 to 2021 in the NPDB reveals a number of repeat offenders: 17,931 physicians with 4 - 10 malpractice payments, 920 physicians with 11 - 50 malpractice payments, and a shocking 40 physicians with greater than 50 payments. While the physicians with over 10 malpractice payments are scary, what's arguably more concerning are the 17,931 physicians with 4 - 10 malpractice payments. In the current system, those physicians can quietly resign from one hospital, move to another hospital or another state, and continue to practice medicine unencumbered.

Is the decline of medical education contributing to the large number of malpractice suits and payments? Evidence from the NPDB suggests the answer is yes. Of the malpractice claims paid out between 1986 to 2010, 28.6% were for diagnostic errors – and 41% of those diagnostic errors resulted in the patient's death. The two main reasons for a diagnostic error are lack of knowledge of all the different possible diagnoses (stemming from inadequate medical school education), or lack of experience in the varied ways diseases can manifest itself in patients (due to inadequate residency training).

Unfortunately, doctors may not readily disclose their diagnostic or other medical errors because they have been brought up in a fail forward model. A study examining how doctors would respond to a hypothetical medical error involving a cancer patient revealed that the majority of doctors surveyed would not admit the error to the patient. The degree of hubris required to withhold the truth from a patient with cancer could only come from someone who has never suffered any consequences for mistakes or subpar performance.

There are even more extreme examples of how doctors in independent practice are allowed to fail forward. "Dr. Death", also known as Christopher Duntsch, was a Dallas-area neurosurgeon who was sentenced to life in prison after numerous patients he operated on were left paralyzed or died. Duntsch had issues throughout his entire medical career, from trouble in medical school to signs of drug addiction during residency. Fellow surgeons who operated alongside Duntsch questioned whether he actually knew anatomy. Despite that, Dr. Death was quietly passed (i.e. encouraged to resign instead of being fired) from hospital to hospital without any mention of serious safety incidents or pending malpractice cases. Two hospitals ended his operating privileges without reporting the inciting reason to the NPDB or to the Texas state medical board.

Although Dr. Death's medical malfeasance could be discarded as a "one off" phenomenon, the story reveals a systemic lack of oversight, as well as a willingness of medical professionals to look the other way when they see a colleague doing something wrong.

Aside from dangerous doctors, the other consequence of fail forward medical education is that there will be more mediocre doctors practicing medicine in the US. And unfortunately, for the average patient looking for a doctor, there is little to no transparency on which doctors provide high quality care. Better doctors don't get to charge more to insurance than their subpar colleagues. Thus, there is no way for a patient to determine the quality of their doctor via price. And publicly available hospital and healthcare organization rankings don't disclose data on the quality of individual doctors.

So how is a patient supposed to figure out whether their doctor is excellent or a dud? It's time to stop idolizing doctors and start scrutinizing them. What I advise is to make friends with nurses who will give you honest information, because there is no way to select a great doctor based on free market information. Do your research before an appointment and ask the doctor questions. A good doctor should welcome questions and provide complete and well-reasoned answers. If your doctor seems miffed that you are even asking questions, that's a major red flag that they are not secure in their knowledge or that they are not used to hearing anything but "yes."

Indeed, today's doctors hear "yes" a lot. As medical students they pass through a school that can only continue to operate if nearly all the students receive a medical degree. When they become residents treating patients the stakes become much higher, but the system's incentives are the same. Residency programs graduate residents to keep their programs running. Learning from those educational experiences, doctors practicing independently perpetuate a culture which is akin to a cabal, with a cultish way of protecting their own.

Knowing the real state of medical education and training should make anyone seeking medical care more skeptical of their doctor. And that skepticism should extend to the functionality of hospitals and healthcare organizations, which mix fail forward doctors with administrators who have been promoted above their level of competence.

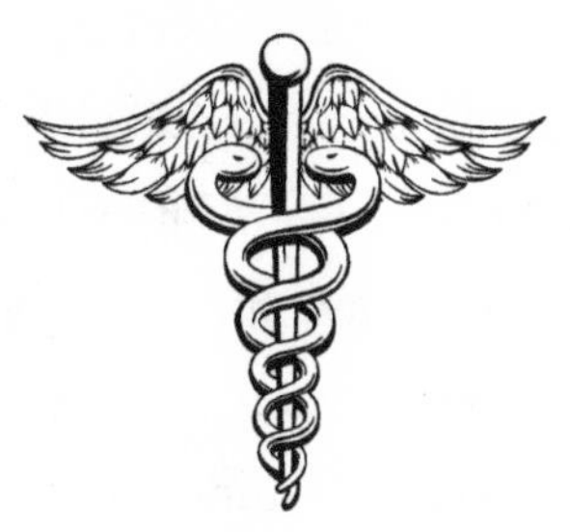

HEALTHCARE ADMINISTRATORS: THE PETER PRINCIPLE

"My first reaction was, 'Which desk jockey sitting at home came up with this nonsense?... The incompetence was just stunning to me. If they had just told us what was going on I would have felt better. But instead they just kept saying we have enough masks.... When this is over, those of us who don't die are going to quit."

—Nurse Kristin Cline, to ProPublica on hospital administrators during the COVID-19 pandemic

"Good followers do not become good leaders."

—Laurence J. Peter

The Peter Principle: Why Things Always Go Wrong

In March 2020, a resourceful intensive care nurse in New Jersey recognized a crisis, rallied her colleagues together, and solved a problem. Olga Matievskaya at Newark Beth Israel Medical Center saw firsthand how the early wave of COVID-19 patients were infecting staff who did not have personal protective equipment (PPE). She started a GoFundMe page and raised $12,000 to buy much-needed masks, shoe covers, and jumpsuits to protect herself and her co-workers.

And what was the reaction of the administrators at her hospital? Rather than thank Olga for her quick thinking and promote her to head of supply chain, hospital administrators suspended Olga without pay for "distributing unauthorized protective gear." Never mind that Olga had won the international Daisy Award for extraordinary nursing in 2019 and her critical care skills were needed more than ever. It was as if no PPE at all was better than PPE bought by staff demonstrating more competence than management.

Olga wasn't alone. Early in the pandemic, nurses across the country were suspended and some terminated for wearing self-purchased PPE or for refusing to work without proper PPE. Ironically, a few months later the same managers who suspended Olga and others turned into the mask-wearing police.

Throughout the pandemic, hospital administrators have continued to make bone-headed decisions. What to do with expired N-95s lying around? Throw them out, of course, until the government publishes studies on their efficacy. What to do when staff get COVID-19? Stay quiet and don't inform workplace contacts who were exposed. Perhaps most alarmingly, what to do about a critical nursing shortage? Fire staff for not taking a COVID-19 vaccine, while simultaneously calling in the National Guard to fill the vacant positions.

How is it that healthcare administrators, presumably dedicated to health and safety, would blindly follow whatever the latest email chain dictated rather than common sense? How is it that after two years of missteps many of these administrators are still employed and pulling six or even seven-figure paychecks?

The answer lies in the Peter Principle, which states that if a worker displays competence in their job, they will be promoted to the next level of management. However, the skills that make one competent at a job do not necessarily translate into being a great manager. The new manager may be less competent, or even incompetent, at his new administrative position, and the promotions will stop there. That phenomenon is often summarized as "people are promoted to a level above their level of competence."

But the Peter Principle applied to medicine is worse. Healthcare administrative promotions are really based on compliance. Therefore, in healthcare, managers can rise a level, or two, or even three, *beyond* their level of competence, so long as they are compliant with whatever instructions are in their email inbox.

And there is an ever-growing pool of healthcare administrators blindly following orders in search of a promotion. Between 1975 - 2010, the number of physicians in the US grew by 150%, roughly in keeping with general population growth. Healthcare administrative positions grew by 3,200%, redefining the meaning of a top-heavy organization.

In the business of healthcare, when that many people rise a level or two above their level of competence, things can go terribly wrong:

During Hurricane Katrina, many hospitals in the New Orleans region lost power and had their backup generators fail due to flooding. That occurred despite having entire offices of hospital administrators assigned to "disaster management." It never occurred to people employed full-time to think about ways things could go wrong in a flood zone to consider that low-lying hospital generators might flood and fail.

Foreshadowing COVID-19, the H1N1 (swine flu) pandemic in 2009 revealed hospital, state, and national medication, mask, and testing swab shortages. Despite after-action reports recommending measures that would have alleviated many future COVID-19 issues, nothing was done.

Aside from disasters and pandemics, individual departments at hospitals waste millions of dollars a year on medical supplies. Hospital administrators fail to stockpile for now routine drug shortages, and at some smaller hospitals, life-saving medications are unavailable for the patients who need them the most. And rather than keep ventilators bought for COVID-19 for future use, instead those ventilators are thrown away.

Don't be fooled into thinking a hospital is any different if it's run by a doctor. Only the most compliant doctors join the C-Suite ranks, including the key Chief Executive Officer (CEO), the Chief Medical Officer, and occasionally the Chief Financial Officer of your local hospital. That last position is truly a disaster, as doctors are notoriously naïve about finance.

COVID-19 has given the public a glimpse inside hospitals' dysfunction. However, most of the inner workings of hospitals, clinics, and entire healthcare organizations are still opaque to those seeking medical care. Therefore, the best way to see the Peter Principle at work is through insider stories of incompetence and dysfunction. These start right at the top with the CEO.

EARLY APRIL 2020

"If this prediction is true (which based upon my epidemiological experience, it is accurate), then we will have a 550% surge in ER volume, and our ICU will be 300% over capacity, by late April."

My heart sank as I read that email from our hospital's Director of Emergency Preparedness. That forecast was apocalyptic. There was no way our hospital could handle that type of patient load. (Fortunately, the early COVID-19 forecasting models grossly overestimated the toll the virus would take. However, none of us knew that at the time.)

"Thanks for the update!"

That was the full reply from our CEO. Not exactly what one would expect, given the current tense atmosphere and the need to plan seriously for an impending viral disaster. However, as I would learn during my time on our hospital's COVID-19 committee, those types of curious replies were the norm.

JUNE 2020

"We've managed to find a dealer for an order of up to 10,000 N95s, however they're all construction-grade N95s and not the NIOSH-certified 1860s that all our staff have been fit tested for. Given the dangers of wearing masks not approved for the healthcare setting, my office will continue in its efforts to procure NIOSH-certified N95s for our staff."

WTF. At that time hospital staff were treating COVID-19 patients wearing flimsy surgical masks. We got one new surgical mask every two weeks and were instructed to store it in a brown paper bag, as if that was some magical sanitizing chamber. Who was this supply chain desk jockey to refuse construction-grade N95s, a massive improvement upon the current situation?

"Great job!"

Again, that was the full reply from the CEO. I imagined him scrolling through emails on his phone, reading the first and last sentence of each, and typing his short replies while he prepared for a guest spot on the local morning news. The local news outlet loved our CEO – he was charismatic and looked handsome in his white coat (the white coat was to remind everyone that he was a doctor, although he hadn't treated a patient in over 20 years). But charm alone doesn't run a hospital, especially during a pandemic.

"The Tent" was the brainchild of our Master of Public Health-trained Infection Control Officer and our Master of Health Administration-trained Director of Emergency Preparedness. Neither had any real clinical experience: Infection Control referenced a mission trip to El Salvador as his medical training, and Emergency Preparedness referenced his military experience (but never said that it was in the Coast Guard). By July 2020, our ER waiting room was packed with a mix of sick people who needed medical care and panicked people who were fine but wanted a COVID-19 test. It was not unusual for the ER waiting room to be chaotic, but during the pandemic administrators actually paid attention to it, and so they decided we needed "The Tent."

The Tent dominated emails and meetings. "*Where should it go?*" "*How big should it be?*" And most importantly, "*What color should we pick?*" Actually, color was an important choice, although not for the reasons the administrators thought. If you're going to do disaster medicine in the summer correctly, you want your outdoor triage tent to reflect the sun. It gets hot in those tents, especially in the summer. Our sage hospital administrators chose a dark navy tent (*"It's similar to the colors of our logo!"*), which absorbed all the heat the summer sun had to offer.

It took one week to erect The Tent in the parking lot, and then it just stood there. The initial planning meetings hadn't involved any of the staff who would work in The Tent (or any of the staff who just lost their parking spots). After two more weeks of Zoom meetings, The Tent was declared operational in the middle of a very humid summer.

Patients still went into the nice, air-conditioned ER lobby to check themselves in. But when they were told to go to The Tent, many refused:

"I walked here from home, I'm not going back outside!"

And from wise African-American patients:

*"What kind of Tuskegee s*** you got goin' on in there?"*

The patients who did walk into The Tent suffered for it. It must have been 95 degrees inside. There was one fan. All the staff were sweating through their PPE and their face masks were perpetually fogged up. Patients with COVID-19 who had fevers fainted from the combination of their illness and the sweltering heat. Techs had to constantly run back and forth from The Tent to the main hospital building for supplies.

Some patients called the local media to complain. They said we were making people sicker in The Tent (true), and that we didn't know what we were doing (very true). Our CEO was quick to send an email about the "extenuating circumstances" in the face of this "unprecedented pandemic," and that everyone, management included, was doing a "heroic job." Still, the Tent came down the next day. However, everyone involved in The Tent's long life of planning and short life of operation still has their job.

APRIL 2020

I was pretty sure I was treating my first COVID-19 patient. It was a young man in his twenties, fresh off the plane from New York City. For the past five days he had fever, chills, body aches, and then started having shortness of breath and difficulty breathing. His chest radiograph looked awful with ground glass opacities throughout his entire lungs. He asked me if he had COVID-19.

"We'll test you and find out."

I should've waited before promising a test. At that time early in the pandemic, all COVID-19 testing had to be cleared by our hospital's public health hero, the Infection Control Director. He insisted we call him to request every COVID-19 test, and the lab wouldn't run the test without his permission.

I paged Infection Control. He called back an hour later.

"Hi there, I've got a young male with all the characteristics of COVID: a week of high fever and flu-like symptoms, and now shortness of breath and pulmonary interstitial disease on his chest X-ray. He just traveled here from New York. I'd like to test him for COVID."

Pause.

"Was he in South Korea, Iran, or China before New York?"

"No."

"Italy?"

"No."

"Then why are you calling me?"

"Because I think he has COVID and I think he needs a test."

"You know our algorithm. We're screening by travel to hot spots."

"Have you watched the news recently?"

"I spend all day tracking the CDC's guidance and reading on-the-ground epidemiological reports. I'm afraid we can't test him. Yes, there are some cases in New York City now, but I'd say it's more likely he has flu than COVID, since he's not coming from those hot spot countries."

"Are you serious?"

"You know, we just can't test everyone that you think has COVID."

"Have I ever called you to request a COVID test before?"

Click.

The patient tested negative for flu. I did everything I could to avoid admitting him because I knew he wouldn't be isolated from other patients. After several hours and multiple respiratory treatments, he was able to breath comfortably without supplemental oxygen. I discharged him with instructions to isolate himself and monitor his oxygen levels with a portable pulse oximeter. I don't know what came of him after that. I do know that a year later our Infection Control Director was promoted to Director of Public Health.

"Hey is pharmacy still here this late at night? I got a question for them about Regeneron."

"They leave at 9 pm, I'll page them for you."

It was late summer 2021 during the peak of the delta wave. I had a patient who was a middle-aged woman with metastatic breast cancer who had caught COVID-19. She met our hospital's criteria for getting Regeneron, a monoclonal antibody treatment for COVID-19. We had been administering Regeneron for several months, and from what I saw first-hand, it seemed to be a great treatment.

It was 8:50 pm, so the phone rang quickly as pharmacy was eager to go home.

"Pharmacy here."

"Hey, there! I'm trying to order Regeneron for a patient in Bed 5, but I can't find it in the EMR formulary."

(EMR stands for the electronic medical record; formulary is the list of available hospital drugs.)

"You read your emails today?"

Since March 2020 reading email communications from hospital leadership was an absolute nightmare. Policies changed several times a day. The tone of the emails went from patronizing to hysterical and now histrionic. The emails themselves got longer and longer, despite being written by people who claimed to be busy 24/7 fighting the pandemic.

"I'm on shift. I don't have time to read my emails."

"We're switching from Regeneron to Bamlanivimab. That's why you can't order Regeneron."

"Ok, how do you spell the new one so I can find it in the EMR?"

"Well, we don't have any Bam yet."

"But we're out of Regeneron?"

"Yes."

"Do we have any monoclonal antibodies?"

"No."

I gave the poor patient in Bed 5 the bad news, then I gave her the state department of health phone number and told her to call in the morning. Hopefully, they would know of another clinic nearby that had monoclonal antibodies.

The next morning our hospital CEO sent a self-congratulatory email bragging about our ability to give patients monoclonal antibodies precisely when we had no monoclonal antibodies in the entire hospital. I got the full story from a nurse my next shift, when we were still waiting for our first shipment of Bamlanivimab.

"Rumor is CEO has a buddy who works for Eli Lilly. Hence, the pressure to use this Bam stuff."

Eli Lilly is the manufacturer of Bamlanivimab.

"Why can't we give both?"

"Well, you know they gave Trump Regeneron, and down in Florida, they're calling the other one 'Ron's [De Santis's] Regeneron.'"

Our CEO really was an aspiring politician.

"And, of course, supply chain couldn't figure out how to ensure we had enough Regeneron until the Bam stuff arrived, right?"

"Of course."

And the patient with breast cancer? She later came back to the ER with shortness of breath and was admitted to the hospital. Fortunately, she survived. Would she have been able to stay out of the hospital if she had gotten monoclonal antibodies? We'll never know.

In case you were hoping that academic medical centers and their doctors were any better, I have another story for you.

Everyone thinks ERs are busiest on Friday and Saturday nights. Not true – it is Sunday and Monday that are the busiest nights. And so one Monday evening I walked into a shift expecting to work hard, but not realizing just how hard it was going to be.

The ER had two "sides." Since this was during my brief stint at an academic hospital, the "A side" had an attending physician, resident, and medical student, and it saw the sickest patients. The "B side" had an attending physician and a nurse practitioner, and it saw lower acuity patients and all of the psychiatric patients (of which there were many). I was scheduled to work the B side. What I didn't realize was that I was also going to be working the A side as well.

An hour into my shift, the A side resident wandered over.

"Hi, I'm Sarah! I'm one of the residents."

"Hi, Sarah."

I turned back to my charting. I already had chemically sedated three psychiatric patients, which requires a lot of documentation.

"I was wondering if you wouldn't mind seeing this asthmatic with me in Bed 2."

I stopped my furious typing.

"Don't you have an A side attending?"

"It's Dr. Waters tonight."

"And?"

Sarah looked uncomfortable. I felt bad.

"As you can see I'm new here, what's up with Waters?"

"He doesn't, you know, doesn't actually see the patients. Bed 2's a child who's pretty sick, and I think they need to go to the pediatric ICU."

I got up and walked with Sarah over to A side. We passed by Dr. Waters at his work station. He looked engrossed in his computer. The Euro Cup soccer tournament was playing on the screen.

Room 2 turned out to be very sick. The patient needed a host of medications and BiPAP (a type of respiratory assistance), which the resident had felt uncomfortable starting by herself on a child.

I left the room and walked over to Waters. He was now shopping for messenger bags – I guess Euro Cup was in a commercial break.

"Hey! I saw Room 2 for you. That kid's gonna need to go to the pediatric ICU, I started him on BiPAP."

Waters looked up.

"Thanks so much, appreciate it!"

Throughout the rest of the shift, Sarah and the medical student would periodically wander over to ask me about patients. My outrage over my colleague's complete abdication of his professional duty was quickly overtaken by my worry about the patients supposedly under his care. Fortunately, I think we managed to get all the patients what they needed that night.

I brought this up to my department chair at the first available opportunity. That would be the first of several meetings and revelations that drove me out of academic medicine entirely.

"Of course, Waters sees his patients, but I'll talk to him about your experience. He also spends a great deal of time in research and medical education. He's very highly ranked by the medical students for giving them autonomy in exploring patient care."

Apparently, "autonomy" meant no supervision whatsoever, and "exploring patient care" meant medical students were in charge of treating the inner-city, uninsured patients who came to our teaching hospital.

I thought the chickens had come home to roost for Waters when he was sued for medical malpractice. A patient he had discharged went home and immediately died of a heart attack. The resident had misread the EKG. Waters had never looked at the EKG (this was during March Madness – the NCAA basketball tournament). Yet our department chair ran cover for him, working to get the suit quickly settled and without any professional consequences for Waters.

The reality was if the department chair fired or disciplined any one of us it would put a political target on his back. He was always at war with the other medical school administrators over budget allocations and couldn't show any weakness.

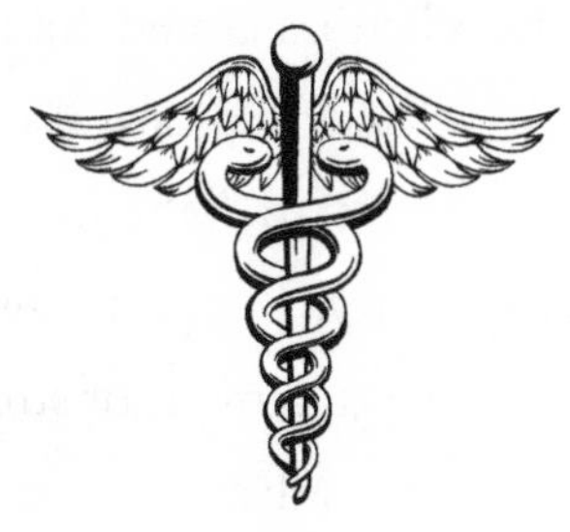

HOSPITALS: FIRST WORLD PARASITES

"A hospital bed is a parked taxi with the meter running."

—Groucho Marx

"The very first requirement in a hospital is that it should do the sick no harm."

—Florence Nightingale

If hapless hospital administrators are products of the Peter Principle, then what keeps hospitals afloat – and proliferating? They must be good at something. As insanely incompetent as they may be at providing actual medical care, hospitals and their administrators are shockingly effective at pushing unnecessary procedures (and some at committing plain fraud) to ensure the hospital's financial bottom line.

Hospitals set prices behind closed doors in collaboration with insurance companies. Hospitals also consolidate into powerful mega-corporations to fight off calls for accountability or price transparency. Hospitals also essentially buy their accreditations for the treatment of strokes and traumas, treatments that help them advertise their costly brand of healthcare.

Rank and file doctors don't push back against this system. Doctors learn in medical school and residency that compliance leads to professional advancement. Like soldiers in today's military, good, hard-working physicians know they will suffer extra scrutiny for speaking out and otherwise displaying independence, while physicians who toe the party line will be left alone or promoted.

All the while, patients are left defenseless and without the practical means to seek personalized, thoughtful medical care.

The epitome of this system are the for-profit hospital mega-corporations. Even if your town still has a local community hospital, it might be owned by a private equity firm, which is even worse. Regardless of who owns them, for-profit hospitals make sure they appear to fulfill all the government's quality of care metrics, while price-gouging their unsuspecting patients.

The most notorious player in this market is HCA, the largest for-profit hospital corporation in the US, with over \$2.3 billion in profits in the third quarter of 2021 alone.

HCA's 163 facilities across the country often do not contain HCA in their names, leaving patients unaware they are seeking care at a controversial for-profit entity. HCA's signature transgression is performing seemingly unnecessary cardiac catheterizations, an expensive procedure wherein a wire is threaded up a patient's femoral artery and into the heart. In some unfortunate cases, HCA patients suffered from near-fatal arrhythmias and cardiac arrest after the catheterization.

Besides risky cardiac catheterizations, HCA's hall-of-fame scandal is $1.7 billion in Medicare fraud, with allegations of direct involvement by then CEO Rick Scott. HCA's board of directors ended Scott's tenure as CEO, but Scott then failed forward into becoming a Florida Senator. HCA was fined and 14 middle-to-upper management sacrificial lambs were criminally prosecuted. But today HCA continues to treat patients across the country because HCA is part of the protected class. Bill Frist, a family member of HCA's founders, ascended to the Senate Majority Leader position in 2003, and therefore it's no surprise that HCA's operations are virtually unencumbered.

But political cover cannot wholly save HCA from bad press. HCA was back in the news during the pandemic when the National Nurses United union filed a complaint with the federal Occupational Health and Safety Administration (OHSA) alleging that HCA hospitals in 17 states were engaged in unsafe practices related to COVID-19. The OSHA complaint alleges staff were forced to come into work at HCA hospitals after testing positive for COVID-19, that staff exposed to COVID-19-positive patients were not notified of the exposures, and that staff requesting COVID-19 tests after exposures were denied testing. One HCA employee succinctly summarized HCA's general operating principles during the COVID-19 scandal: *"We know nurses will be positive [for COVID-19], so we're not testing them."*

It's not just HCA. Tenet Healthcare, another major for-profit hospital corporation, had one of their California hospitals raided by the FBI as part of an investigation into 769 potentially unnecessary heart surgeries and associated Medicare fraud. Tenet wound up paying $900 million in fines to Medicare, but no fine can undo invasive surgeries performed on patients.

But it's not just HCA and Tenet. Policies and procedures at hospitals and clinics across the country push unnecessary medical procedures. From pelvic exams to screenings for cervical cancer in low-risk women, to imaging scans that expose patients to radiation, to needle pokes for blood work, hospitals leave no stone unturned in their search for higher reimbursement from insurers. And they receive no pushback from the compliant doctors who are told to order the tests. The waste and potential for medical harm, even for low-risk procedures, is staggering. A single study from Washington state estimated 600,000 patients in a single year were subject to an unnecessary medical procedure. Another study in

Virginia estimated that $586 million was spent annually on unnecessary medical care.

So beware of a surgeon asking if you'd like your daughter's ears pierced while she's under anesthesia for a surgery. That ear piercing will cost thousands of dollars and not be covered by insurance. Also beware the latest fancy medical technology, as this is another ploy to drive up costs and hospital profits. The President of the Association of American Physicians and Surgeons in 2018 admitted as much, *"One of my patients received an invoice of around $100,000 for a hysterectomy, of which $68,000 was for the use of a robot."*

And while most doctors comply with hospital policies that push unnecessary procedures and inflated bills, the imposition of electronic health records on all medical institutions by Obamacare makes it easy to police the remaining rogue, independent doctors. Open the electronic chart for a patient who has chest pain, and automatically an alert pops up prompting you to order a chest radiograph and an electrocardiogram. If you try to ignore that alert (say the patient just has really bad acid reflux causing chest pain), the computer will ask for a justification. Even if you justify your "inaction," that alert will continue to pop up over and over again until you finally submit.

Unfortunately, non-profit hospitals in the US aren't any better than the for-profit hospitals. In fact, non-profit hospitals may be better at gaming the system than their for-profit colleagues, since non-profit hospitals enjoy federal tax-exempt status valued at $24.6 billion.

In exchange for giving up the capitalist dream of profits, non-profit hospitals are supposed to provide charity care to uninsured and very poor patients. Charity care should mean billing discounts and flexible payment plans. In practice, however, charity care isn't charitable. Applying for charity care is incredibly difficult, as evidenced by one hospital's application that included questions about the make and model of the patient's car. By not approving charity care applications, non-profit hospitals can send patients inflated bills devoid of any discounts. Since those bills are impossible to pay, many non-profit hospitals now have their own collections agencies to chase down poor patients.

The aggressive billing and collections practices of non-profit hospitals don't result in money invested back into services for patients. Quite the opposite. While not paying federal taxes, non-profit hospitals funnel revenue in excess of expenses into 7-figure executive pay, bonuses, lavish conferences, private jets to fly to those lavish conferences, and even offshore bank accounts. What happens when non-profit hospitals engage in blatant, egregious, and repeated practices that run contrary to the spirit of their non-profit tax-exempt status? Nothing. Unless you count sternly worded letters from Congress that lead to no punitive action.

Are there any standards that hospitals are held accountable for? Yes, the nonsensical healthcare metrics of the US federal government. That is because the Centers for Medicare & Medicaid Services (CMS) is the biggest insurer in the US, with Medicaid and Medicare covering about 40% of Americans. Because CMS has the business obligations of an insurer and the power of the federal government, its interest in healthcare standards doesn't translate to better patient care – it means that one of its main goals is to decrease expenses. CMS uses its metrics to justify paying healthcare organizations pennies on the dollar or for denying reimbursement outright.

Since losing payments, however small, for almost half of your customers and invoking the ire of the federal government is never good for business, hospitals are held captive by CMS's Quality-of-Care metrics. Those metrics are a compilation of mortality, safety of care, timely and effective care, hospital readmission rates, and a patient experience survey called the Hospital Consumer Assessment of Healthcare Providers and Systems (HCAHPS – pronounced "H Caps"). If you're multitasking reading this book and looking up your local hospital, you'll see if the hospital is below, the same, or above the national average, and how many stars your hospital got out of a possible five. However, the reality is that healthcare administrators manipulate the CMS metrics, and some of the metrics themselves are flawed.

For example, while mortality could be a legitimate metric, hospitals can game it by keeping vegetative patients alive just past the due dates of their CMS reports, and then pull the plug on life support afterwards.

Also ripe for manipulation using the electronic health record is the timely and effective care metric. For example, CMS measures how quickly ER patients are seen by a doctor. The solution for that is a click button on the computer screen indicating, "Medical Evaluation Initiated." Simply place your mouse cursor over the patient's name, right click, and win CMS points! As many hospital administrators will emphasize to their staff, reading a patient's name on the computer screen constitutes initiating the patient's evaluation.

CMS also measures the number of ER patients who leave without being seen by a doctor. That metric is harder to game, but it can be done. Crafty ER's set up systems called "doc in a box," or "triage doc," where a doctor literally sits in a closet briefly examining patients who are in the ER waiting room, ordering tests and scans. That way if an ER patient leaves after waiting for hours, the hospital can, somewhat truthfully, claim that he didn't leave without being seen by a doctor.

CMS's Quality-of-Care metrics also include hospital readmission rates. This is measured as an unplanned readmission within 30 days of a first admission. On the one hand, hospitals and doctors should do their best to discharge patients only when it's safe to do so. However, not all patients are angels. Some patients don't take their medications, or fail to go to follow-up appointments, and end up back in the hospital. Sometimes, despite following medical advice, patients get worse. Doctors and hospitals know that they will be "dinged" by CMS for a readmission ("dinged" is hospital slang for lower reimbursement). That perversely incentivizes hospitals to do everything in their power to not admit patients who are failing outpatient management and need to be hospitalized. CMS' readmission penalties also make doctors hesitant to promptly discharge patients to their homes for fear they will "bounce back" and be readmitted.

And is the HCAHPS patient experience survey any better of a metric? Unfortunately, no. HCAHPS surveys patients after they have been discharged from a hospital admission, but the very first problem with the HCAHPS survey is how it is administered. Hospitals self-administer the survey and self-report their results to CMS. That alone could lead to some bias. But even worse, the actual practice is for hospitals to pay consulting firms to administer the survey for them. The incentive for the consulting firms is to give hospitals good results, thus making the hospitals happy customers who keep hiring the consultants. To do that, consulting firms solicit numerous HCAHPS surveys and then cherry-pick the best ones to report, since CMS only requires a certain number of surveys to be reported each year

What does the HCAHPS survey measure? Most questions ask patients how well their doctors and nurses communicated with them during their hospitalization. Nothing wrong there. However, some now-retired HCAHPS questions may have helped fuel the opioid epidemic. Prior to 2019, the HCAHPS survey asked questions about pain, specifically how often was pain well-controlled, and how hospital staff responded to and managed patient's pain.

In this author's opinion, those questions incentivized hospitals and doctors to administer opioids to gain favorable HCAHPS survey responses. A common scenario went like this: a patient is in pain after surgery to remove their appendix. The patient asks for pain medication. The patient's doctor remembers the slew of emails from hospital administrators advising that the hospital needs to be responsive to patients' pain, because HCAHPS scores last year were less than stellar. Consequently, rather than start first with less-powerful, non-opioid painkiller and see whether the patient responds, the doctor immediately orders a powerful opioid, ensuring favorable HCAHPS responses. And unfortunately, when opioids are given to patients in the hospital, it's likely that opioid prescriptions will be written for that patient when they are discharged home. After all, it's unreasonable to expect someone to be comfortable taking over-the-counter ibuprofen at home after they've received powerful intravenous opioids for the past few days in the hospital.

In a classic case of "thou doth protest too much," the Journal of the American Medical Association published a study denying that HCAHPS pain scores were associated with more opioid prescriptions. However, while publicly denying a link between HCAHPS and opioid prescriptions, the American Medical Association's (AMA's) friends at the American Hospital Association (AHA) quietly lobbied CMS to drop the pain questions from HCAHPS.

CMS finally removed the controversial HCAHPS pain questions in 2019. In this author's opinion, personal experience, and reported experience of colleagues, the HCAHPS pain questions absolutely did increase opioid administrations in the hospital setting, which inevitably resulted in more opioid prescriptions at the time of discharge, and thus many new tragic opioid addictions.

Does CMS really care about patients so much that they spend all that time and effort compiling these Quality-of-Care metrics? Of course not. The real purpose for CMS' metrics is to justify the government's Value-Based Purchasing (VBP) program, which CMS uses to haggle with hospitals over reimbursement. VBP allows CMS to justify paying pennies on the dollar for Medicaid and Medicare patient charges. All CMS needs is a hospital to score low on some metric and suddenly a $10,000 charge from the hospital to CMS becomes a $200 bill from CMS to the hospital.

CMS also wields the VBP program to enforce the federal government's political goals. During the COVID-19 pandemic, as part of the Coronavirus Aid, Relief, and Economic Security (CARES) Act, CMS gave hospitals a 20% add-on to reimbursement rates for Medicare COVID-19 patients who were admitted to hospitals, regardless of the actual reason for admission. That created two dangerous incentives. One, it incentivized the admission of COVID-19 patients who perhaps could have perhaps been discharged home. Two, the 20% COVID-19 add-on incentivized the reporting of asymptomatic COVID-19 patients who sought care at hospitals for unrelated conditions, like mental health problems or broken bones.

Regardless of the intent, Medicare's COVID-19 20% add-on program drove hospitalization rates of patients suffering from and suffering with COVID-19 higher. And now as the government begins to pivot away from the never-ending COVID-19 saga, the VBP program is being wielded to enforce social agendas. Starting in 2022, doctors will receive extra CMS reimbursement if they create and implement an anti-racism plan.

"Patient relations is coming over to see you."

"Oh no, what did I do?"

"They said they're bringing over a patient."

Another reason I prefer working nights shifts over day shifts. At night management is home in bed and can't interrupt clinical care. I quickly hid the coffee and snacks that I'm not supposed to have in the ER.

Patient Relations strutted into the ER in her high heels and skirt suit. Accompanying her was a mother who pushed her school-aged daughter in a wheelchair. The girl appeared to be developmentally delayed.

"We've had a bit of an incident in the main hospital lobby, I was hoping you could help."

Patient Relations had vague down to an art form. She probably drafted our CEO's emails.

"I can try but I'm going to need to know what happened."

"Yes, yes, of course, can we go to a private room?"

"Are they checking in as a patient?"

"Well, no, maybe you can just examine the daughter first."

Perfect. The hospital screwed up and we want you to fix it, but of course we're not going to follow the proper procedure. Instead, we're going to ask you as the ER doctor to assume personal liability for a "curbside consult." (A curbside consult is when a doctor informally gives their medical opinion.)

I turned to the mom and asked what happened.

"We were in the lobby waiting to visit my father, who is in the ICU. I can't believe that your hospital, which is ranked highly in the US News and World Report rankings, decided to decorate for the holidays with Poinsettia plants, which are poisonous! My daughter has cerebral palsy and she ate one of the plant leaves and now is having an allergic reaction."

I turned to the daughter. The area around her lips was red, and her lips were slightly swollen. Other than that, she didn't look to be in any distress. Still, potential angioedema (swelling of the lips, tongue, and airway) is nothing to mess around with.

"Yes, they are poisonous, though not as deadly as you think. Still, anyone can have an allergic reaction. Let's get her checked in as a patient so I can properly examine her and order some allergy meds."

Patient Relations looked displeased. Her carefully constructed world of patient satisfaction scores was being blown apart that morning. While the triage nurse was measuring the girl's vital signs, Patient Relations turned to me and huffed:

"In the future, be careful with how you use the term poisonous."

"Poinsettias are technically poisonous, though you'd have to eat 500 leaves to die. What you really should be concerned about is the oleander shrub out by the front entrance. That thing can actually kill somebody. (All parts of the oleander plant contain a cardiac glycoside, which can be fatal if ingested, even in small quantities.) *And don't ask for my medical opinion if you don't want it."*

"When you're done, make sure you apologize to the family for the hospital."

Patient Relations strutted out, her high heels making strange noises on the dirty linoleum ER floor.

The redness and swelling went away with some Benadryl. I put the mom on the phone with Poison Control, who reassured her the daughter was going to be all right. The mom asked me if she should file a formal complaint. I told her yes, absolutely.

Beyond gaming CMS's quality of care metrics, hospitals also obscure their inner dysfunction by advertising misleading awards and accreditations. If you have ever searched the internet for hospital rankings, undoubtedly you have come across the *US News and World Report* "Best Hospital Rankings." For decades *US News and World Report* has controlled the hospital rankings game, which are medicine's equivalent to the Oscars.

But what if you searched for your local hospital in the Best Hospital Rankings and didn't find it? You're not alone. To be eligible for the medical Oscars, a hospital must be a teaching hospital, or affiliated with a medical school, or have at least 200 beds, or have at least 100 beds and 4 "advanced technological capabilities." By *US News and World Report's* own admission on their website, about half of the country's hospitals are eligible for their rankings. So if you live in a rural area or are a veteran using the Veterans Affairs system, tough luck.

In addition to ranking hospitals overall, *US News and World Report's* Best Hospitals ranks hospitals by medical specialty. Here, too, there is another important exclusion from the rankings – the commonly needed specialties of primary care and emergency medicine. Two of the most frequent means by which someone encounters the medical system are curiously absent from these supposedly all-encompassing rankings.

Now that we know who is eligible for the medical beauty pageant, what exactly do the rankings measure? Best Hospital Rankings combines metrics which are similar to CMS's Quality of Care metrics with a survey of doctors' expert opinion.

The expert opinion poll is controversial because it is wholly derived from a survey that asks doctors to name the five best hospitals in their specialty. (Also worth noting is that three specialties' rankings rely solely on the expert opinion survey: ophthalmology, psychiatry, and rheumatology). Even if doctors were to respond truthfully to the survey, it would result in impractical advice for patients. For example, an oncologist would likely name the largest and most prestigious cancer centers the country has to offer. But it's well out of the means of most Americans to fly far away from home for cancer treatment.

However, most physicians do not respond to the expert opinion survey truthfully. Annual emails from the C-Suite and patient relations give the marching orders: 1) Fill out the damn survey, 2) Get 3-5 of your colleagues to fill it out too, and 3) Of course you know that your hospital is the best, right? In fact, some hospitals employ teams of analysts dedicated to gaming the annual *US News and World Report* rankings. Often they work side-by-side with the analysts dedicated to gaming CMS metrics. Not surprisingly, the rich, brand-name hospitals flush with analysts win the rankings game year after year. Meanwhile the poorer, smaller, more local hospitals fall in the rankings, tarnishing their reputation, and lowering their sticker price for the inevitable opportunistic buyout by a large hospital corporation or private equity firm.

[Author's note: I'm good friends with a hospital clerk. This is her story as recounted to me.]

As a clerk I'm supposed to answer phones, send and receive paperwork, help get the doctors and nurses what they need, and of course help patients with whatever I can. Yet lately all I'm allowed to do is be a sitter for the psychiatric patients. The ER is overflowing with suicidal and psychotic patients, and someone has to sit and watch them 24/7 to make sure they don't take the hospital sheets and hang themselves or strangle someone else.

I was mid-way through one of those "reassigned sitter shifts" watching five psych patients at once when all hell broke loose. A little old African-American woman who insisted she was George Washington called a white meth head a "cracker." The meth head yanked the oxygen port fixture out of the wall and started hitting George Washington over the head with it. I was the only one around, mind you, so I quickly backed up towards the door and yelled for security. It took three security guards to separate them (George Washington was feisty), and the doctor had to order lots of chemical sedation that was injected into the patients' thighs.

Only after things calmed down did the ER charge nurse appear. Rather than ask me if I was OK and talk about how we could make this situation safer, she asked, *"You finish the Mock Joint Commission staff survey yet?"*

At the beginning of the shift, she had given me a paper survey to complete in preparation for our Joint Commission accreditation. The mock surveys were used by hospital management to identify "trouble areas" to clean up just before the Joint Commission survey team arrived to inspect the hospital in person.

"Did you not hear what just happened here? No, I have not filled out the survey yet."

"I need it by noon."

She left. I sat down and looked at the survey, glancing up every few moments to look at the psych patients, who seemed woozy, for now. I started laughing. The survey had questions like: "On a scale from 1 - 5, how safe do you feel at work?" and "On a scale from 1 - 5, how much do you feel that your supervisor cares for your well-being?"

As I went down the list of questions, my laughter turned to anger. I had no formal training to deal with psych patients. I wasn't getting paid extra for these reassigned sitter shifts. I had heard there was a Botox clinic out in the suburbs looking for a receptionist. Surely that was better than this.

So I circled one, the lowest ranking, for all my responses.

The charge nurse returned, and I handed her the survey. George Washington and the meth head had both woken up and were starting to trade insults again.

"Did you mean to circle all fives instead of ones?"

"No, I meant to circle all ones."

"We can't turn in this survey. You're going to have to redo it."

"It's a mock survey."

"This is preparation for the real Joint Commission visit."

"Ah I see, this is practice for me to lie."

"No, we don't want you to lie. If you have any concerns, you can always bring them to me."

This from the charge nurse who was always absent when there were any problems that needed fixing.

"You can fill the survey out for me. I'm not feeling well today. I'm leaving."

I got up from my chair and walked out, just as George Washington and the meth head started fighting again.

Aside from gaming metrics and rankings, hospitals buy accreditations for treating conditions like strokes. Billboards conveniently placed on the highway an exit or two before the hospital proclaim, "Comprehensive Stroke Center" or picture an elderly man clutching his chest to show that you that heart attacks are cared for off Exit 12. But with how accreditations really work, the average patient has no way of determining whether they are walking into the best stroke center in the world, or a hospital that excels at filling out paperwork.

What does it mean to be a "Comprehensive Stroke Center"? Surely if a hospital was not an actual stroke center, some plaintiff's attorney would sue for false advertising. It turns out there are a variety of ways to truthfully proclaim you are an accredited stroke, or heart attack, or whatever type of center.

For example, in the case of stroke centers, there are multiple types of accreditations, all ending in the designation of being an accredited stroke center. The Joint Commission (an Orwellian-named, supposedly independent organization that doles out accreditations and reports back to the government), has four levels of stroke accreditation: comprehensive stroke center, thrombectomy-capable stroke center, primary stroke center, and acute stroke ready hospital. A hospital with any one of those four levels of accreditation will proclaim on billboards that it is accredited to treat strokes. However, avoid a "stroke ready hospital" if one side of your face is drooping, because that designation really only means the ER staff should be able to recognize a stroke.

It turns out The Joint Commission is a customer-pleaser that acts with accreditations just as consulting firms do with the HCAHPS survey. In fact, The Joint Commission advertises on its website that, *"We certify 10 times the number of Acute Stroke Ready Hospitals as the competition."* That claim reveals the business model of The Joint Commission and other accreditation companies: charge hospitals application fees, and in return, accredit as many hospitals as possible.

And who are the competition The Joint Commission mentions? It turns out hospitals unwilling to engage with The Joint Commission can easily turn to other accreditation companies with an easier process or less expensive fees. Regardless of the accreditation organization, it all results in the same highway billboard declaring, "We're a Stroke Center!"

How lucrative is the accreditation racket? It costs tens of thousands of dollars, per hospital, per year, to pay for the accreditation review and on-site visit. That fee doesn't include the hundreds of thousands, if not millions of dollars spent on full-time employees dedicated to re-certifying the accreditations. Like CMS metrics and Best Hospital Rankings, here too hospitals have teams of analysts dedicated to keeping up appearances. So not only is the accreditation process costly, but it also contributes to hospitals' administrative bloat.

But even lack of accreditations doesn't stop hospitals from engaging in misleading advertising. Perhaps you've seen a highway billboard with a cute child playing soccer with the tagline, "We Care for Kids!" What does "We Care for Kids" mean? Absolutely nothing. That hospital could be a world-renown children's hospital with every pediatric subspecialty.

Or that hospital could be a small community facility with no pediatric staff, and one room in the ER dedicated for pediatric patients because the television is set on the Cartoon Channel. The dishonest advertising of pediatric services may be the most amoral and egregious example of hospitals gaming the system to gain patients. Parents of a sick child are not typically in a calm, rational state of mind to be able to research whether a hospital truly can "care for kids."

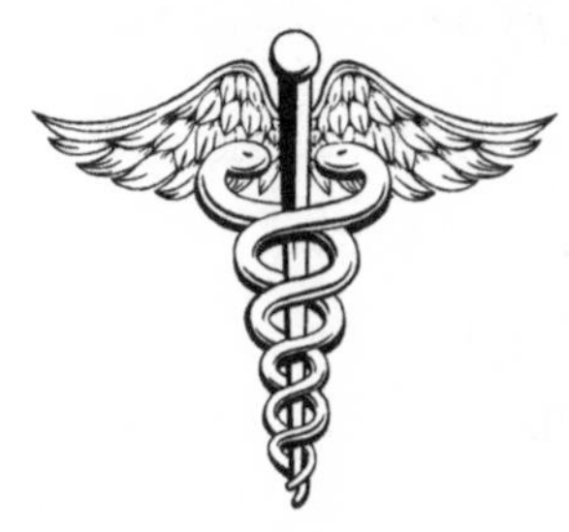

MEDICAL PROFESSIONAL SOCIETIES: THE SKY IS LAVENDER!

"Achieving health equity is not a utopian dream."

—American Medical Association
Advancing Healthy Equity: A Guide to Language, Narrative, and Concepts

"Professing themselves to be wise, they became fools."

—Romans 1:22

"Can you come take a look at Bed 7?"

Whenever a nurse asks you to look at a patient, you must do so, immediately.

"Is Bed 7 getting their blood transfusion now?

"Yup, he doesn't look so good. I mean, she's not feeling well."

Bed 7 was a patient who was biologically male, but had transitioned to being female. She also had Crohn's disease and was in the ER tonight for a flare, with severe abdominal pain and bloody diarrhea. Her hemoglobin was dangerously low from her gut not absorbing iron and from the blood loss. We were giving her a blood transfusion prior to admitting her to the GI service.

I walked into the room and instantly saw it was bad. The patient was breathing heavily, sweating, and looked even more pale than when we started the transfusion. Even though blood banks go to extensive lengths to match blood donors to patients, there is still the possibility of a transfusion reaction. With the patient's difficulty breathing, I was worried about transfusion-related acute lung injury, which can be serious, even fatal.

"Stop the blood, give 50mg of IV Benadryl and 1,000mg IV Tylenol. We'll have to draw the transfusion reaction labs and let blood bank know."

After the patient was stabilized, I got on the phone with the blood bank.

"We had a transfusion reaction and are sending you the reaction panel labs. It was a male-to-female transgender patient with Crohn's disease and..."

The pathologist cut me off.

"Wait, did you say male?"

"Yes, male-to-female transgender."

Silence on the other end of the line.

"But the electronic medical record says female."

I questioned myself for a second. It was my fourth shift in a row. I pulled up the patient's chart in the electronic medical record. Yup, sure enough, on the big, highlighted column with patient demographic information it said male under "sex," and female under "gender identity." The hospital recently had upgraded the electronic medical record to a new version that included the gender identity label.

"We sent you blood matched for a female patient. When I looked at the chart all I saw was female and a female name, I didn't see the male sex."

Uh oh. Blood transfusions are sex-matched because of an increased risk of a transfusion reaction if a male receives blood from a female. And now this patient was having a transfusion reaction.

Fortunately, the patient recovered. However, the hospital and electronic medical record's hurried adoption of a new virtue-signaling gesture without consideration of the unintended consequences could have killed the patient – the very type of patient such gestures are advertised to help.

In fact, the ensuing hospital safety committee "after action" meeting revealed who the new gender identity label was *really* meant to help – hospital administrators in their careerist pursuit of following progressive dogma. Each administrator made a habit of beginning his presentation with a preamble like: *"We all agree it is vitally important to support our transgender patients,"* and *"Of course, we all agree it is imperative to display someone's gender identity loud and clear in the electronic medical record."*

The clinical matter at hand was that we'd given a patient the wrong type of blood, and our mistake had led to a serious and potentially fatal transfusion reaction. But since the long-winded virtue signaling took up the entire meeting, that matter was never addressed.

A few months later our hospital received a designation as a "Leader in LGBTQ Healthcare Equality" from the Healthcare Equality Index.

The truth is that major medical professional societies have always had progressive goals and embraced governmental authority, so it is hardly surprising that medicine has joined other industries headlong rush to "wokeness" and politicized the business of healing patients. That said, it is one thing for medical societies to toe the political line and proclaim, "The sky is lavender!", but quite another for individual doctors to subordinate patient health to sociopolitical goals.

Unfortunately, that's where we find ourselves, with innumerable doctors falling into lockstep with the dictates of medical professional societies, including what biological science is permissible to believe and what treatment options should be available to patients.

That was made crystal clear during the COVID-19 pandemic when drugs were all but labeled with (R) and (D) political affiliations (a.k.a. ivermectin and Remdesivir). And decades of disguising social engineering as the science of public health have produced new MPH-certified "healthcare heroes" who preach on social media about guns as a public health problem and fat acceptance (because criticism of obesity is racist).

Yet most of the time those politicized actions backfire, to the detriment of patients. That is why I hope those on the left side of the political spectrum are still reading this book, because presumably when they seek care as a patient, they are looking for medical advice, not a summary of *The New York Times'* opinion column.

The bottom line is you can't just listen to your doctor anymore without judging their words in the same way you would in listening to a political commentator. And if a "prestigious" medical society endorses a policy or a treatment, you should be skeptical of the immediate effects on your health and the secondary effects on healthcare.

The statements and actions of the American Medical Association (AMA) illustrate how most medical professional societies are political in nature. Indeed, the AMA has been a progressive pit bull for over 150 years. The AMA was founded in 1847 to represent doctors and publish the *Journal of the American Medical Association* (*JAMA*), now one of the most widely read peer-reviewed medical journals. Although the AMA's mission purports to "promote the art and science of medicine and the betterment of public health," it really is focused on the second task. And as we have seen recently, public health is really the government extending its reach further into individuals' private lives.

Early AMA actions included lobbying for more government regulations in the Drug Importation Act of 1848. Under the guise of filtering out poor-quality medicines from Europe, the Drug Importation Act restricted overall drug supply in the US If you are still waiting for ivermectin tablets to arrive from India months after your original online order, you can trace your difficulties back to the AMA.

It is not surprising that the AMA would advocate for more government regulation of what drugs individuals might procure for themselves. Looking at over 100 years of advertisements from the AMA's journal *JAMA* reveals a heavy bias towards pharmaceutical company interests. Some early *JAMA* pharmaceutical ads were so blatantly misleading that the broader 19th century progressive reform movement briefly turned on the AMA. The AMA's misstep had revealed its allegiance with big pharma.

Playing defense, in 1905 the AMA and *JAMA* began a voluntary program requiring drug companies to show proof of their claims in advertisements (i.e., display data from clinical trials conducted by the drug companies themselves).

That voluntary program made the AMA look once again like model citizens to progressives, and it got ahead of new laws passed by Congress in 1912 that made false claims of drug efficacy a criminal offense.

Yet, as we see with COVID-19 emergency use authorizations and FDA drug approvals today, the definition of efficacy is always up to the government, receiving cherry-picked data from pharmaceutical companies. Medical organizations will follow suit and assist with disseminating the agreed-upon talking points around "efficacy." In the case of the AMA, whatever drug or vaccine is deemed best by the government will be championed by *JAMA*. The converse is also true – whatever therapeutic regimen is associated with political enemies will be thoroughly condemned and repudiated.

The recent case of Remdesivir and hydroxychloroquine illustrates how the AMA and *JAMA* throw their prestige around in service of political goals. A *JAMA* review in April 2020 treated both drugs fairly in describing their relative risks and benefits, including side effects, costs, and availability. Then President Trump casually but favorably mentioned hydroxychloroquine in May 2020, sparking an immediate backlash against the generic drug. *JAMA* then ran an editorial on the "Misguided Use of Hydroxychloroquine for COVID-19," which cherry-picked research studies that concluded hydroxychloroquine was not efficacious in treating COVID-19, while failing to mention studies that showed benefits. Yet *JAMA* has yet to run such an editorial highlighting the bad outcomes and side effects from the brand name drug Remdesivir.

However, even before COVID, in 1966 President Lyndon Johnson was alarmed by inflation and the rising price of eggs. He ordered his Surgeon General to highlight eggs' "health hazards" to decrease demand for the breakfast food staple. *JAMA* assisted by publishing a research paper concluding that a healthy diet should not contain more than four eggs per week, and it printed an editorial describing egg yolks' vibrant color as "betraying the offending cholesterol." And there you have the origin of decades-old medical dogma that "eggs are bad for you."

The AMA's love of governmental authority knows no bounds, and includes advocating for compulsory vaccines, from smallpox vaccinations in 1899 to COVID-19 vaccines today. After ignoring first amendment rights to religious exemptions from vaccination, the AMA sequentially tramples through the Bill of Rights to the second amendment. The AMA has repeatedly pushed for gun control, declaring "gun violence" a "public health emergency," coupled with the clichéd petition for "commonsense reforms such as expanded background checks." Typical of its nanny state mindset, the AMA does not believe a grown adult can knowingly consent to engage in any vice whatsoever. The AMA's "war on smoking" has included supporting complete bans on tobacco advertising and increasing cigarette taxes.

To better work in concert with the government, the AMA has its own political action committee, the American Medical Political Action Committee (AMPAC). AMPAC was wooed by Ronald Reagan and briefly opposed Medicare expansion (he did rescue those medical students in Grenada after all!), but AMPAC's statements, and more importantly, monetary political contributions, have always been biased to the left. That leftward push occurs whether or not most of the AMA's members are supportive. For example, AMPAC lobbied hard for the passage of Obamacare, even though most doctors are either opposed to or lukewarm towards the Affordable Care Act.

Despite the disconnect with the members it purports to represent, the AMA today doesn't bother to hide its political bias. Their 2020 Advocacy in Action report called for the Trump administration "to address the conditions of facilities at the southern border" for "undocumented persons' health." The report concluded with a tone-deaf and self-congratulatory summary of its efforts at "addressing health equity," "opposing Medicaid work requirements," "enhancing access to care," and "collaborating with...other like-minded organizations."

While the Advocacy in Action report reads less like medical guidelines and more like cable news talking points, the AMA's 2021 resource guide, Advancing Health Equity: A Guide to Language, Narrative, and Concepts, reads like a contemporary university sociology curriculum. That document insults all the minority groups it purports to support by turning into a parody of itself, beginning with its "Land and Labor Acknowledgement." As it turns out, the AMA's beautiful suburban Chicago headquarters was once the land of indigenous tribes. While the writers "mourn the loss of lives" that "were forced out by colonization, genocide, disease, and war," make no mistake - this pricey real estate is not going to be given back.

The AMA's Advancing Health Equity resource guide goes on to propose an entirely new long-winded medical vocabulary that removes problematic words such as white and black. One wonders whether the white matter in our brains will have to be renamed, and whether the grey matter is safe too.

All joking aside, the resource guide's suggestions and beliefs are already being incorporated in some medical school curricula. If that trend spreads to all medical schools, instead of a fail forward system where students are at least being taught medicine, we will have a fail forward system where cardiology is replaced with critical race theory.

All this begs the question - does the AMA speak for the majority of doctors? As of 2016, the AMA's membership was 235,000, comprising only about 17% of all US doctors. By contrast, in the 1950s fully 75% of US doctors were AMA members. However, the medical students graduating now and in the future will likely align more with the AMA's progressive goals and be more inclined to join the organization.

And like any political movement, more members translates into more financial and political power.

That is a scary prospect, as the AMA's policy advocacy already is strikingly effective, and its legislative victories have limited patients' options for primary care. The AMA used AMPAC funds and cynically leveraged the public's general high regard for doctors to defeat dozens of state bills that would have expanded the scope of clinical practice for nurse practitioners. Those bills would have allowed nurse practitioners to operate more independently, thus increasing the supply of clinical providers and their available time to see patients. The AMA's rationale for fighting the bills was that nurse practitioners are not doctors. What the AMA ignored was that nurse practitioners help alleviate workforce shortages in primary care (especially in rural areas), lower healthcare costs, and provide much-needed competition to the current cabal of doctors.

Unfortunately, the AMA successfully convinced many state legislators that because doctors spend more years training than nurse practitioners, doctors therefore must be more competent. However, as we have already demonstrated, all that time in education and training doesn't filter out bad doctors. The truth is, nurse practitioners (and physician assistants) threaten the monopoly of physicians who want to spend their time rallying for political causes rather than focusing on treating patients.

While the AMA claims to speak for all doctors, individual medical specialties have their own professional societies as well. To best illustrate the strains of political progressivism that run through those specialty organizations, we have the innocent-looking pediatricians from the American Academy of Pediatrics (AAP). The AAP's virtue signaling starts with its motto, "Dedicated to the health of all children." A stickler for grammar and concise writing would note that "Dedicated to the health of children" says the same thing. The purposeful insertion of "all" is meant to indicate that the AAP is especially concerned with children they believe society has marginalized.

Indeed, the AAP's recent "Blueprint for Children" covers topics ranging from immigrant child health to racism. On that latter topic the AAP considers itself a pioneer: *"As we noted in a* ***landmark*** *[emphasis author's] statement on the Impact of Racism on Child and Adolescent Health in August of 2019…"* Whether left- or right-leaning, I doubt any reader would consider a statement on racism circa 2019 to be landmark. The rest of the AAP's Blueprint is filled with buzzwords like food insecurity, gun violence, and climate change. The AAP also craves recognition as a MoveOn-style influencer and organizer, publishing its own "Advocacy Training Modules."

All those documents are utterly devoid of pediatric medicine, but when it comes to medical care, AAP pediatricians reveal themselves to be far left. In a 2016 resource document co-published with the Human Rights Campaign

Foundation, the AAP advocated for an affirmation approach towards transgender children. The affirmation approach includes supporting social transitioning (e.g., manner of dress, school bathroom of choice, changing gender and name on birth certificates), and gender transitioning (e.g., prescribing puberty blockers and cross-gender hormone therapy, and referral for gender reassignment surgery).

The AAP's stance on pediatric transgender issues brought attention to a much smaller, conservative pediatric society called the American College of Pediatricians (ACPeds). ACPeds quickly released a statement declaring, *"Facts - not ideology - determine reality."* Conservative commentator Glenn Beck tweeted about the ACPeds statement and featured a commentary on his website implying that a major pediatric professional society had equated promoting gender dysphoria with child abuse.

The echo chamber on right-wing cable news ran with the story, except that they and Glenn Beck got a key detail wrong. ACPeds is *not* a major pediatric society, but rather a small, alternative, even fringe, medical professional society. As left-wing media outlets were quick to point out while defending the "prestigious" AAP's affirmation approach, the ACPeds has barely received any prior recognition and has no historical clout in medicine.

The spat between right- and left-wing pediatricians echoes society's general political divide, with leftist organizations dominating headlines and fundraising while right-wing organizations play catch-up. The extent of the AAP's political clout was made apparent when Hillary Rodham Clinton appeared as the keynote speaker for their 2014 national convention. Never mind that in the same year her policies as former Secretary of State helped unleash a civil war in Libya that proved disastrous for children in that region, the YouTube video of Clinton's speech shows adoring pediatricians looking upon an idol as she downplays the role of family in raising children:

> *"I want to spend my time today talking with you about this life-changing work. Because it is to me so self-evident...that when parents...turn to for an answer about their baby, hands down...it is their pediatrician. I can tell you that answer is now, far ahead of, oh, my mother. Eventually we get back around to my mother, but we start with the experts."*

As organizations like the AMA and AAP run amok, their talking points filter down to individual physicians. Those physicians, blithely assured that they know what is best for the world, have become fanatical and narcissistic. Society's long-standing admiration for doctors probably inadvertently contributed to those in the medical profession having such an inflated sense of self. Little wonder that as the COVID-19 pandemic took hold, so many doctors seamlessly assumed the mantle of authority figures on television, social media, and in real life. Our new #HealthcareHeroes overnight became

Twitter-certified epidemiologists and Instagram PPE models who moralized, “We stay here for you, please stay home for us.”

The media followed suit and lionized the new public health apostles. Typical of the glowing media spotlight was a Vice News segment on a Los Angeles ER doctor “struggling” during the virus’ second wave. Intended to serve as a grave warning to non-medical personnel to lockdown their own lives, the video attempts to paint this doctor as a secular saint nailing herself to a cross. Yet to those of us who have actually treated COVID-19 patients, the Vice News video is pure comedy. The segment opens with the ER physician donned up in her PPE talking somberly about the waves of bodies crashing upon the ER (never mind that she somehow has plenty of time to talk to a reporter…). Then comes the obligatory scene where she removes her PPE, finishing by taking off her N95 mask and gasping for air (it’s not *that* hard to breathe through a N95, trust me). If you feel bad for this lady, that quickly fades as you watch her escape the ER by driving off in her Tesla.

Of course, during a pandemic the “doctor-as-hero” analogy is not always fraudulent or exaggerated. But the post-shift selfies comparing creases on faces from N95s to the plight of a soldier at war were ridiculous and offensive. In the US, at least, no one was fighting COVID-19 at gunpoint. Moreover, any doctor who’d read medical history would know full well that serious pandemics arise every hundred years or so. Once-a-century apocalyptic events aside, there are many other well-known hazards of being a physician. However, there are no Instagram stories or Tik Tok videos about occupational exposures to other deadly diseases like tuberculosis or HIV.

Not sensing how ridiculous the #HealthcareHeroes movement was, the social media posts from doctors were invariably devoid of any irony or self-awareness. To underscore how all-consuming and exhausting it must be caring for COVID-19 patients in the ER and ICU, doctors and nurses began making TikTok videos with choreographed dances in their PPE and Tyvek suits. Because nothing says, "This disease is so terrible, and we're totally overwhelmed!" as turning the ICU into a scene from *High School Musical.* Gallows humor has its place, but watch some of those videos and think of the time that must've gone into their production – time that could have been spent trying to wean sick COVID-19 patients off the ventilator (or avoiding using a ventilator in the first place).

All this overshadows the real healthcare heroes who have been around long before COVID-19: combat medics and Doctors Without Borders. The heroism of combat medics needs no explanation. Doctors Without Borders physicians dodge bullets in Congolese war zones while treating simultaneous outbreaks of COVID-19, Ebola, and measles. Beyond risking losing their lives to infectious diseases, physicians from Doctors Without Borders have been abducted from the Congo and shot while in Afghanistan.

But even being #HealthcareHeroes isn't enough for doctors, who are also embracing the role of victim by promoting "physician wellness and combating burnout." Those buzzwords have become a convenient excuse for medical errors, failing board exams, and other displays of poor performance.

In 2021, the Federation of State Medical Boards and the National Board of Medical Examiners announced that the Step 1 United States Medical Licensing Examination would become pass - fail. Step 1 is the first of the three general US medical board exams and is taken after the second year of medical school. A student's numerical Step 1 board score used to be heavily weighted in their residency application. No longer. Now all residency programs will see is a pass or fail, and medical students get six tries to pass. What's the cited reason for that change? Physician wellness and burnout. Now we see that doctors' obsession with their own well-being has lowered standards for everything from board scores to treating COVID-19 patients in the ICU.

Did doctors suddenly become tone-deaf during the pandemic? No – the disappearance of doctors' humility and its transformation into an enhanced sense of self-importance is a result of the confluence of falling educational standards and the public health movement. The inclusion of public health in the practice of medicine has tipped the balance over to where generally speaking, for obviously there are exceptions, doctors' sense of self-importance knows no bounds.

Today the field of public health is touted as a science, but it's really an excuse for government action in the pursuit of an unattainable utopian society. Public health's more legitimate accomplishments (e.g., the epidemiologist Jon Snow discovering the source of a cholera outbreak in London in 1854), have dissipated in favor of schoolmarm safety rules. Examining the CDC's top ten list of public health accomplishments shows a move away from combating deadly infectious diseases to policing activities that are best described as under the purview of individual choice (e.g., smoking, seatbelts, and bike helmets). Now post-COVID-19, whatever the progressives need to satisfy their agenda, or whatever the government needs to gain more control, is justified in the name of public health.

Yet many of public health's crowning achievements have had unintended consequences or even outcomes that ran counter to the stated goal. Sunscreens that were supposed to prevent skin cancer contained carcinogens. The fluorine added to our drinking water and toothpaste to prevent tooth decay is linked to thyroid problems. The Chantix drug prescribed to people who want to quit smoking so they don't get lung cancer turned out to have an ingredient that can cause cancer!

Yet despite those and other massive failures, the field of public health is undeterred. Persistence in the face of obvious evidence to the contrary can only come from the siloed halls of academia, and here we have the Master of Public Health (MPH) graduate programs to thank for the public health disciples chanting for pandemic lockdowns.

Looking at the MPH curriculum for the oldest school of public health in the US, the Harvard T.H. Chan School of Public Health (yes, here too the Chinese are funding the West's decline), reveals the extent to which public health has migrated from infectious disease containment to social engineering. The classes for the two-year generalist MPH degree read like a television lineup for *PBS* or *MSNBC*: "Human Health and Global Environmental Change," "Narrative Leadership – Using Storytelling to Mobilize Collective Action in Public Health," "Health Equity and Health Justice: A Global Perspective," "Social, Behavioral, and Structural Determinants of Health," and the *Rules for Radicals*-inspired "Public Health Policy and Politics" and "Communicating for Impact in Public Health."

In two full years of public health study only one required class touches on biostatistics and quantitative methods. Yet as you may have seen on social media or heard on the news, MPH-decorated public health figures like Rochelle Walensky at the CDC feel capable and empowered in interpreting the complex biostatistical methods of today's big pharma clinical trials. Doctors like Walensky have no business even speaking of the methods of a clinical trial, let alone interpreting whether the results are statistically or clinically significant.

Perhaps the most dangerous combination of medical training today is the combined MD-MPH. Medical schools let students fail forward while reciting progressive medical society talking points, and public health schools teach that what constitutes medicine includes surveilling whether citizens are wearing face masks.

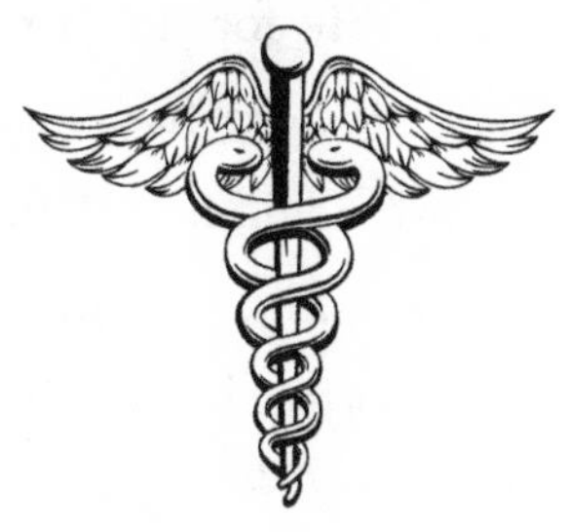

HEALTHCARE INSURANCE: TOO BIG TO BARGAIN WITH

"The financial crisis is a stark reminder that transparency and disclosure are essential in today's marketplace."

—Jack Reed

"Hospitals and commercial health insurers keep the rates they privately negotiate confidential for good reason: it would undermine competition if they were required to be disclosed publicly."

—American Hospital Association

Michael Flor awoke from a medically induced coma in the intensive care unit at Seattle's Swedish Issaquah hospital. His last memory was 29 days prior, saying goodbye to his wife over the phone, presumably for the last time before being intubated. Against all odds, he had survived even though his lungs and kidneys were failing due to COVID-19. Staff dubbed him the "Miracle Child." Yet Michael was wiser than a child, telling his wife shortly after waking up, *"You gotta get me out of here, we can't afford this."*

Michael Flor had health insurance, yet his 181-page hospital bill still came to a grand total of $1,122,501.04. Since Michael was an early survivor of severe COVID-19, his bill went viral and many of the charges magically disappeared. However, other patients hospitalized later in the pandemic were not so lucky. Without high-profile news coverage there wasn't any pressure on healthcare insurers to drop outrageous charges. And as the number of hospitalized COVID-19 patients grew, somehow those patients' bargaining power shrank.

During the pandemic, many people were scared and sought COVID-19-related testing and treatment regardless of their insurance status. One would think that waves of pandemic-related claims would cause healthcare insurance companies to buckle under the financial pressure. The insurance situation seemed akin to what happens after a natural disaster, as in 1992 when Hurricane Andrew bankrupted many property insurers following payouts totaling $15.5 billion. But unlike then, today there are no small to medium-sized health insurance companies running on real profit and loss statements. What we have instead are corporate goliaths reaping record profits, all with the backing of the federal government. Sound familiar?

Healthcare insurance companies today are like the Big Banks circa the 2008 financial crisis. Healthcare insurers are too big to fail, and thus they are protected and supported by the federal government. And just like the Troubled Asset Relief Program pretended to regulate banks while solidifying their power over the economy, Obamacare's supposed regulations for healthcare insurers have reinforced their strength. With the healthcare insurance mandate, Obamacare created a captive customer base for the healthcare insurance companies.

Also similar to the stress test and reserve requirements that became mandatory for financial institutions post-2008, there are now so many government regulations for healthcare insurers that smaller insurers simply cannot survive. It is only through vast resources and economies of scale that the big insurance companies stay afloat.

For example, Obamacare's prohibition on considering pre-existing conditions when pricing or offering healthcare insurance plans was a death sentence to smaller insurance companies. For a healthcare insurance company to remain financially viable, there must be a certain ratio of healthy people paying premiums while not using services to offset the sick people in the insurance plan who need healthcare. Large regional or national insurance companies with millions of enrollees have the financial buffer to remain viable in an environment where insurers cannot turn away or charge high premiums to patients with pre-existing conditions. In other words, only a large company that can sustain a quarterly loss or two can survive in today's twisted healthcare insurance market. Whatever small insurance companies were left after the passage of Obamacare in 2010 were bought out by large insurance companies who saw an opportunity to further consolidate power via horizontal integration.

But even before the Affordable Care Act passed, another little-known fact that contributed to the death of small to medium-sized healthcare insurance companies was the reinsurance market. Most insurance companies *reinsure* themselves against significant losses (whether small quarterly losses or catastrophic pandemic losses). Actuaries for reinsurance companies pick the long-term winners and losers, and thus smaller firms were priced out of existence due to unaffordable reinsurance premiums.

All this relates to private insurance companies. But what is the situation with government-run insurance plans? It's important to underscore that through the Centers for Medicare and Medicaid (CMS) the US government is the biggest healthcare insurer in the country. Medicare and Medicaid have nearly double the number of enrollees of the biggest private insurer, UnitedHealthcare Group. Theoretically, the US government could regulate their competition, the private insurers, out of business. That would make some progressive politicians very happy. But rather than compete, the relationship between government and private insurers is symbiotic. Private healthcare insurance companies are one of the biggest government donors. In return, the government allows private healthcare insurers to get away with all sorts of anti-competitive practices.

Indeed, private health insurance companies are not satisfied with just horizontal integration. Those insurers realized that Democrat politicians would run cover for them to preserve Obamacare's "legacy," and that Republican politicians would back corporate actions in the name of the "free market." That political environment allowed healthcare insurance companies to vertically integrate.

What does vertical integration mean in the health insurance context? First, it leads to a process of controlling costs and services offered upstream through the purchase of hospitals, clinics, and entire healthcare organizations. Next, it means controlling downstream consumer spending by buying pharmacies and pharmacy benefit managers. Does this sound like a healthcare monopoly? It is in practice, and with all the negative consequences for consumers. Nonetheless, the Department of Justice blessed a $69 billion merger between Aetna and CVS health, which combined clinics, pharmacies, insurance, non-medical retail, and pharmacy benefit managers into one giant conglomerate.

Thus, in addition to competition-stifling regulation, the US government allows giant healthcare insurance companies to become too big to fail. In return, insurance companies donate copious amounts of money and occasionally rescue the government from its more embarrassing episodes – as when a subsidiary of UnitedHealth Group named Optum helped to fix the disastrous Obamacare website. This produces a revolving door between insurance executives and government administrators. That was seen when UnitedHealth Group senior executive Andy Slavitt later became acting administrator for CMS. It also ensures the government's laws and policies remain friendly to healthcare insurers.

Thus, the environment today is similar to the lead-up to the financial crisis of 2008, with the government turning a blind eye upon the predatory actions of healthcare insurers. But it's likely the government will be fully at attention when insurance companies sometime in the future inevitably claim they need bailouts, either due to COVID-19 or some other disaster. After all, by 2026, $1 in every $5 spent in America will be spent on healthcare. How is that not too big to fail?

But being too big to fail isn't enough, as insurance companies also engage in backdoor dealings with healthcare organizations and hospitals to fix prices.

Your health insurance dictates where you can receive healthcare. The place where you receive healthcare charges your insurance company. Herein lies the dilemma for insurance companies: they refer customers to healthcare organizations for medical services, but then they themselves, the insurers, must foot the bill. Surely there must be a better way? Fortunately, the MBA grads at insurance companies have found a solution which guarantees the corporations win and the patients lose: the healthcare organization discounts its charges to the insurance company, and in exchange, that insurance company agrees to not send its customers to competing healthcare organizations.

But what about doctors who wish to practice independently while still letting patients use health insurance? The MBA grads have devised a solution for that too: bills from large healthcare organizations separate facility fees from physician fees, and facility fees are much higher than physician fees. That effectively prohibits independent doctors from working with insurance companies, because doctors working for the large healthcare organizations are comparatively cheaper. Insurance companies simply won't pay independent doctors a higher price than the artificially low prices set by their collusion with healthcare organizations.

To illustrate how this works in practice, let's say you get a nasty cut while opening a package from an online retailer. You go to the hospital, the doctor spends 30 minutes stitching you up, and you spend a total of two hours in the ER. For that visit, the hospital charges a facility fee of $3,000 ($1,500 per hour) and a flat physician fee of $125. Now say the ER doctor who treated you becomes disillusioned and seeks to strike out on his own in independent practice. He wishes to charge a flat rate of $200 for house calls to stitch patients up (a fair market rate for an hour of an ER doctor's time). If patients of this independent ER doctor want to use their insurance, they will simply be denied. *"$200 per hour is more than $125,"* the insurance company will say. *"You must go to the ER at our preferred hospital...which we just bought."* Therefore, in practice, the separation of facility and physician fees and the resulting price distortion prevents the development of a competing system with independent practitioners.

As physician fees are set artificially low, healthcare organizations and insurers can come to a gentlemen's agreement on facility fees, which generate the real profits for both parties. And since hospitals have relatively cheap physician labor and insurers are selling a government-mandated product, both parties have plenty of margin to make a profit. The price fix is simple: healthcare organizations set their minimum acceptable reimbursement from the insurance company, and insurance companies set their maximum allowable charge from the hospital. Somewhere in the middle lies the facility fee. This step is even easier if the healthcare organization and insurance company are both owned by the same parent company – i.e., vertically integrated. It's much easier to quietly collude when everyone is on the same side.

Integral to the hospital-insurance gentlemen's agreement is price discrimination based on insurance type – the better your insurance, the more you will be charged out of pocket. By getting good health insurance, you are signaling to all parties involved that you have more disposable income to drain. If you have Medicaid or no insurance, assuming you somehow manage to get healthcare, you can be charged less because the expectation is there is no way to squeeze water from a stone. In fact, the best thing to do after a major surgery or ER visit may be to feign bankruptcy.

I once found myself at a Christmas cocktail party with a several economists in attendance. I was minding my own business, enjoying the free food, when a friendly man asked me what I did for a living. When I replied I was a doctor, it was as if I set off a magnet that pulled in the economists. Naturally they all were very interested in how their economic theories held up in the real world of healthcare.

I regaled them with a few funny patient stories until one man wearing a bow tie interrupted, *"How many of your patients don't have insurance?"*

"I'd say it's 40% private insurance, 40% Medicaid and Medicare, and 20% no insurance."

"You accept that many people without insurance?"

"Oh yes, the hospital loves them."

"What?"

"We prefer those without insurance to the Medicaid and Medicare patients for sure. Nothing's as good as the private insurance though, because we charge them the most."

Another man opined, *"Of course, this is robbing Peter to pay Paul."*

"Yes, in what's billed to insurance, of course. But the out-of-pocket charges to patients with private insurance are more than what's charged to patients without any insurance."

The original inquisitor sounded offended, *"You must be mistaken!"*

Gotta love it when economists say that you're mistaken about your own profession.

"Listen, as you all well know, hospitals and private insurance companies fix the charges and payments between each other. Medicare and Medicaid pay pennies on the dollar, so the hospital just accepts that those patients are near total losses. You're correct in that the more uninsured patients we see, the more the overall system costs are carried over to private insurance prices. But what you're missing is that the bill to the actual patient with private insurance for the same service will be higher than what we bill to someone with no insurance."

Silence and blank stares. I could sense the beginnings of the academics' cognitive dissonance meltdown and so I simply couldn't help myself from pressing further.

"I'll give you a real-life example. A friend of mine who's another doc broke her arm. She has great insurance. She went to the ER, pretended she was unemployed, and told them she didn't have health insurance at all. They worked out a payment plan with her at 0.5% interest and removed the entire facility fee because they assumed there was no way she could pay it. She ended up paying $500 plus a little in interest for an ER

visit with X-Rays and getting a splint. She's real thorough and estimated that if she used her insurance, it would've been $1,000 in out-of-pocket costs."

One by one the economists awkwardly walked away, some muttering about my "anchoring bias" and "behavioral bias."

Has the US government tried to do anything about the collusion between healthcare insurers and hospitals? Yes – much to the delight of the lawyers representing all parties. In 2019, the Trump administration's Health and Human Services (HHS) proposed a rule requiring hospitals to publish prices they privately negotiated with insurers for 300 common healthcare services. The proposed rule was shocking for two reasons: 1) It required some degree of price transparency in an industry where prices are virtually unknown to patients, and 2) The rule in and of itself acknowledged the collusion between hospitals and insurance companies.

Not surprisingly, healthcare organizations and insurers fought back. Hospitals and other medical interest groups banded together and lawyered up. The American Hospital Association (AHA), the AAMC, and several carefully chosen hospitals sued HHS.

That suit filing is a master study in corporate entitlement and the elite's contempt for the average American. The AHA and the other plaintiffs in the case claimed we plebes do have the right to know how much things cost. But because healthcare costs are such a complex and "multi-stakeholder" process, our simpleton brains could not digest the meaning of prices. Therefore, the lawsuit's argument goes, hospitals could never just put prices on a menu the way a restaurant does (ignoring that restaurants also deal with supply chains and multiple stakeholders).

Boldly, the AHA lawsuit plainly acknowledges the collusion between hospitals and insurers:

> *"The Final Rule requires each hospital in the nation to publicize on its website a huge quantity of confidential pricing information reflecting individually negotiated contract terms with all third-party payers, including all private commercial health insurers."*

The AHA and plaintiffs then go on to conclude that their First Amendment rights as corporations would be violated by publishing prices:

> *"The Final Rule also runs afoul of the First Amendment, because it mandates speech in a manner that fails to directly advance a substantial government interest."*

Since when did posting prices constitute "mandated" speech? Conversely, when did the right to deceive patients by omitting prices become a free speech right? Entertaining the logic of the AHA's argument for one moment, it *is* in the government's interest to know healthcare prices because the government foots the bill for Medicaid and Medicare patients. The lawsuit then goes on to state that widespread knowledge of prices would undermine free-market competition:

> *"Hospitals and commercial health insurers keep the rates they privately negotiate confidential for good reason: it would undermine competition if they were required to be disclosed publicly."*

Read that statement again. The lawsuit argues that if consumers knew the price of a good it would disrupt the classical principle of supply and demand. You don't need an economics degree to realize that statement is ridiculous. But the hospitals and insurance companies think you will believe it:

> *"What patients care most about from a pricing standpoint when selecting a hospital: their own out-of-pocket costs."*

That last statement is factually correct but misleading. A patient's out-of-pocket costs are related to what is charged to his insurer and his type of insurance. The price of a cup of coffee is directly related to the price of coffee beans. However, coffee drinkers can look at posted coffee prices and decide whether to buy cheap gas station coffee or a latte made by a barista. Hospitals and insurance companies have such a low opinion of patients, their customers, that they think patients will buy their laughable assertion that it's better to *not know* the price of their medical care.

A judge also found those assertions laughable and the AHA lost the lawsuit. HHS's price transparency rule became effective in January of 2021. By 2022, however, only 14% of hospitals had complied. And hospitals who did comply used search engine de-optimization tools and other tricks to hide their price webpages from search engines. That outcome makes it plainly obvious that even the legal system poses no real obstacle to the collusion between insurers and healthcare organizations.

Given that the government allows private insurance to freely engage in unethical and anti-competitive business practices, you may be wondering how government itself runs its own healthcare insurance plans, Medicaid and Medicare. After all, those two insurance plans cover nearly half of Americans. If you are guessing that Medicaid and Medicare are run inefficiently and dramatically limit healthcare options, you are correct. What you might not have guessed is that the government's love of surveillance has now extended into Medicaid and Medicare.

To illustrate that we have Accountable Care Organizations (ACOs) – a product of the Affordable Care Act and a great example of utopian ideas on paper that don't pan out in real life. In an ACO, a group of doctors, nurses, and healthcare administrators get together and theoretically coordinate to lower costs while delivering a higher quality of patient care. In reality, ACOs ration healthcare while invading a patient's privacy. Although there are no "death panels," ACOs are a terrifying yet predictable consequence of government overreach.

Let's walk through how an ACO works using an example CMS highlights on its website – the Keystone ACO. This ACO uses "predictive analytics" to flag patients as risks for running up healthcare costs. A "community health assistant" then halts any independent progress that patient has made in taking ownership of their health. The assistant gets to snoop around in the patient's medical chart (without the patient's consent), visit the patient's home, and then develop a care plan. That assistant, assigned by hospital administrators and not selected by the patient, is now the gatekeeper for the patient's access to all healthcare that the ACO will cover. Want to see your family doctor about something sensitive, like erectile dysfunction? You'll have to tell your new health assistant first. Having sudden chest pain and worried it's a heart attack? You are still free to go to the ER, for now, but be aware your assistant might flag that visit in the system as unnecessary, affecting future co-pays and out-of-pocket costs.

The logistics and ethics of ACOs are an obvious nightmare. But fortunately, the government can't even execute rationing properly. One-quarter of patients on government-run insurance plans are in an ACO, but the total annual cost savings to taxpayers in 2017 was $300 million… out of trillions of dollars in expenditures.

With big healthcare organizations and insurers blatantly engaged in business conspiracies, the average individual fraudster feels emboldened. And it shouldn't be shocking given the current state of medical education to learn that some doctors fancy themselves masterminds. And with the health insurance market skewed towards low reimbursements for individual doctors, what is an entrepreneurial doctor to do if he wants to build a water park in the Dominican Republic?

One answer is to bill for numerous medical services, beating lower reimbursement prices (especially from Medicaid and Medicare) by sheer volume. While it's tough to get away with doing lots of unnecessary tests and procedures, those practices don't seem unnecessary once a doctor has "upcoded" the patient's condition. Upcoding involves stretching the truth about the severity of a patient's condition, and it's routinely used by doctors and hospitals alike to fight for higher payments.

Say a patient has mild asthma – there's a specific diagnosis code for that. But if the patient is instead coded as having moderate or severe asthma (different diagnosis codes), now follow-up office visits, pulmonary function tests, and allergy tests are reimbursable events that can be billed to insurance. However, since making repeated clinic visits is time-consuming, and after multiple procedures a wary patient might start to ask questions, unscrupulous doctors can play it safe by doing invasive, costly procedures once; or better yet, by engaging in phantom billing for made-up visits, procedures, and even imaginary patients!

The scope of healthcare fraud is massive. In fact, the FBI has entire teams devoted to healthcare fraud (including a very busy field office in South Florida, always the hub of bizarre criminal activity). And insurers know full well they are being continually bled dry by fraud. In the case of Medicare, the physicians who are billing outliers are well-known and even publicized. Yet while the FBI and Department of Justice focus their energy on political persecutions, the field officers tasked with reigning in healthcare fraud end up playing an endless game of whack-a-mole.

I once had to have a simple outpatient procedure done to remove a benign cyst on my neck. I thought the removal could have been done under local anesthesia, but my doctor insisted I have some sedation so I wouldn't move. I should've known better, but I trusted my colleague, and so I was scheduled to have moderate sedation by an anesthesiologist for the procedure.

Since anesthesia was involved, the whole ordeal had to happen in the operating room. I arrived at my scheduled time, 5:30 am, and changed into the standard flimsy hospital gown. It was freezing in the pre-op room. A nurse asked if I'd like a warm blanket. *"Sure, thanks,"* I replied. She quickly grabbed a blanket out of the warming machine and handed it over.

The procedure was quick, although it took me twice as long to recover from the sedation. My doctor gave me the recap while I was still woozy in the recovery unit. *"Simple excision, simple cyst, minimal blood loss – very easy actually. If it wasn't on your neck, I bet you could've done it yourself! Anyways, come see me in seven days to have the stitches taken out."*

A few months later I received my bill. I was out-of-pocket \$500 for a "complex cyst removal" and \$250 for a "warmed hospital blanket."

In the rigged healthcare insurance market littered with fraudulent practices, what is an individual patient with a chronic condition or true medical emergency left to do? Even the most meticulous and cost-conscious patient can get stuck with surprise and inflated bills.

God forbid you are in a serious car accident. A bystander calls 911 and the ambulance arrives to take you to the ER. From an insurance standpoint, that ER is either in-network or out-of-network. Even if you're conscious and your condition is stable, you do not always get to choose the ER to which you are transported. If you are traveling out of town, perhaps the ambulance takes you to the closest ER, which could be out of network. If you are close to home, but your condition is severe, the medics will likely bypass the closest ER for a trauma center. (Hopefully, the trauma center accreditation is real). That trauma center may or may not be in your network. The resulting surprise out-of-network bills are shocking, with sky-high out-of-pocket costs that leave many patients with little recourse other than to bargain for repayment plans or deal with collections agencies.

Nor is it just ambulance rides and medical emergencies that result in surprise bills for insured patients. Say you need your gallbladder removed. It's not urgent, and you do everything by-the-book, double-checking with your insurance company that the hospital and surgeon are all in-network. Recovering sans gallbladder, you receive a terrifying bill for the anesthesiology services. It turns out, due to weird vertical and horizontal integration patterns and outsourcing, the anesthesiologist who put you to sleep was an out-of-network contractor filling a staffing shortage. You didn't get to pick the anesthesiologist, you met him on the morning of surgery to say hello and consent for anesthesia. What you didn't consent for was the outrageous out-of-network surprise bill.

It's not just anesthesia though. Many hospitals outsource various services. It's everything from radiology to emergency medicine that are staffed by independent contracting companies which may or may not be in-network. A 2010 study found one-third of ER visits and one-quarter of hospital inpatient admissions triggered some type of out-of-network charge. In particular, the ER is fraught with surprise billing traps, as around two-thirds of ERs are staffed by independent contractors. It's impossible to check before you experience severe chest pain whether your ER doctor or the radiologist reading your chest X-Ray will be in your insurance network.

And surprise bills don't stop with out-of-network charges. In an example of just how uncaring healthcare can be, a couple in New York was charged $257,000 out-of-pocket for obstetric and neonatology services after their prematurely born daughter died. The healthcare insurer, Cigna, maintained they'd overpaid the hospital in error, and so they were billing the devastated parents for Cigna's own mistake.

The original sin causing all this mess was tying healthcare insurance to employment. Until the presidency of Franklin Roosevelt, most Americans paid fee-for-service for the healthcare they received, and employees in high-risk occupations like coal mining had access to employer-sponsored clinics for the treatment of occupational hazards and diseases. So how did we get from there to mandated healthcare insurance and nearly half of Americans on a government-run insurance plan? It was FDR's 1942 Stabilization Act that radically altered the US healthcare insurance landscape.

Outwardly, the Stabilization Act had nothing directly to do with healthcare. Theoretically, it was designed to prevent wartime inflation from turning the US into Weimar Germany. In addition to a host of price controls set at FDR's discretion, the act limited the ability of employers to raise wages to compete for workers. Now unable to compete for scarce workers based on salary, employers had to get creative to attract workers, and so they expanded employer-sponsored benefits, including employer-sponsored healthcare.

Although intended to be temporary, the new trend of employer-sponsored healthcare insurance was made more attractive in 1954 when the Internal Revenue Service made employer contributions to health plans deductible expenses for the employer, and tax-exempt income for the employee. The lingering question of how retirees and unemployed Americans could obtain healthcare insurance was "solved" in 1965 when President Lyndon Johnson created Medicare and Medicaid.

Thus, a little presidential meddling in the economics of inflation created by printing money to finance a war turned into a dysfunctional marriage of healthcare insurance to employment and the creation of two permanent and ever-growing government programs.

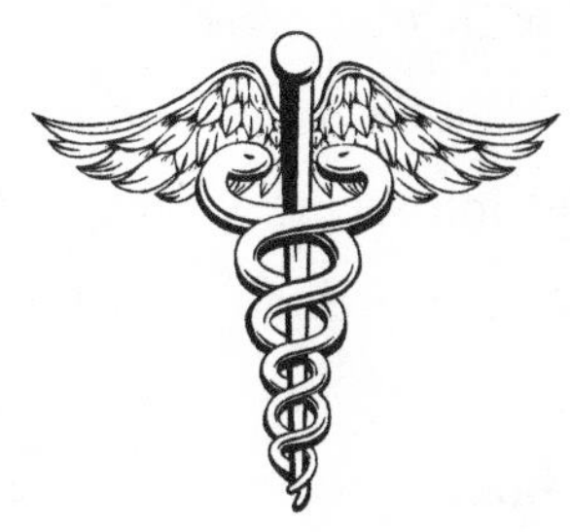

THE CDC & NIH: A JOBS PROGRAM FOR BUREAUCRATS

"Bureaucrats complicate. It gives them more work to do. It gives them job security. It means promotions as ever more bureaucrats are added to the Ministry of Redundancy."

—Sieg Pedde

Although both the Centers for Disease Control and Prevention (CDC) and the National Institutes of Health (NIH) had broad name-recognition prior to the COVID-19 pandemic, currently not a day goes by without major news coverage of both agencies.

But stepping back – where did the CDC and NIH come from and how did they come to play such an important role in American healthcare?

Post-World War II, there was a glut of wartime offices filled with recently deputized bureaucrats who now needed a new purpose, and job security. Hence, like our military, government healthcare agencies like the CDC and NIH were either founded or saw their power grow tremendously during the post-war baby boom years. Over the next few decades, the military mindset of one-size-fits-all orders combined with popular culture's worship of scientific advancement created an environment where agencies like the CDC and NIH flourished, at least on paper.

Today, in the wake of COVID-19, it's become obvious to millions that things have gone so terribly wrong at the CDC and NIH that those agencies are more apt to create problems rather than solve them. In fact, a knowledgeable observer will make the case that both the CDC and NIH have been dysfunctional from the outset, and indeed, that the problems they create while 'solving' other problems are a feature rather than a bug.

Quite simply, if you're a bureaucrat, whether at the Pentagon or at the CDC, your existence depends upon a steady supply of problems to ensure Congress lavishly funds your livelihood. Thus, when one problem is "solved," another *must* be created. And in the never-ending fight for more government funding, the bigger the problem, the better. Mere problems do not attract nearly as much funding as crises – like a war or a pandemic.

Seen in this way, the CDC's and NIH's response to COVID-19 represents not a breakdown in government agency function, but a continuation of the status quo.

The fact is both the CDC and NIH have demonstrated incompetence throughout their *entire* existence. As those agencies became more powerful and better funded, in some respects our health declined and our healthcare system steadily became worse at its actual job: healing patients.

Talking heads on television make the CDC sound like it has been a vigilant public health watchdog since the American Founding, protecting colonists from malaria in the swamps of Virginia and Oregon Trail settlers from giardia in mountain lakes. The Hollywood image of the CDC is one of nerdy doctors in hazmat suits protecting Americans from hot zone diseases, like Dustin Hoffman in the movie *Outbreak* (although Dustin Hoffman's character actually worked for the United States Army Medical Research Institute of Infectious Diseases).

In actuality, the CDC is filled with more off-the-rack suits than hazmat suits. The CDC is no different than any other government agency started in the aftermath of WWII – the agency is a way to make permanent an enormous wartime government and provide job security for loyal bureaucrats.

The CDC grew out of a 1946 merger between the US Public Health Service (PHS – founded during the late 19th century progressive political movement) and the military's WWII Malaria Control in War Areas program (supported by the Rockefeller Foundation). Thus, the CDC's origins were progressive, militaristic, and globalist, and had nothing to do with protecting stateside Americans from disease.

Headquartered in the natural swamp of Atlanta, the CDC made its first mission to protect US citizens from malaria. It's a disease caused by a parasite, and humans are infected via mosquito bite. However, the malaria eradication program was executed not with traditional medical "first do no harm" ethics but rather with wartime scorched earth tactics.

The CDC used its first annual budget in 1947 to spray as much land as possible with the chemical dichlorodiphenyltrichloroethane (DDT). DDT is very effective at killing mosquitos, but it also kills wildlife, contaminates crops, and can cause cancer in humans. DDT's potential lethal effects were overlooked, as only seven of the original 369 CDC employees were medical doctors. After blasting southeastern farmland with a crop-killing carcinogen, the CDC declared its first major public health victory – eradicating malaria from the US in 1951. However, the CDC never bothered to collect short-term or long-term data on the unintended consequences and secondary effects of its widespread DDT use.

After defeating malaria, the CDC needed a new mission to justify its annual budget, and so the agency moved on to syphilis by assisting with the Tuskegee Experiment. To grasp the sheer evil of this atrocity perpetuated against thousands of African-American men, their sexual partners, and their children, a brief primer on syphilis is required.

Syphilis is a sexually transmitted disease caused by a bacteria called *treponema palladium.* Syphilis in its initial, primary stage causes localized disease in the genital area of the infected individual. However, left untreated, primary syphilis progresses beyond a localized infection to the entire body, which is known as secondary syphilis.

Both primary and secondary syphilis can be readily treated with the antibiotic penicillin. However, untreated secondary syphilis will become latent (i.e., hidden) in the body. In some latent cases, the syphilis bacteria later awaken and invade the brain, nerves, eyes, heart, liver, and other organs. That condition is known as tertiary syphilis and can cause dementia and death (historical note – Al Capone died from complications of tertiary syphilis). Additionally, syphilis is easily transmitted between sexual partners, and babies born to mothers with syphilis suffer from congenital syphilis, a horrible, irreversible condition causing deafness, facial and tooth deformities, and even premature birth or stillbirth.

Ostensibly to better understand this horrible disease, in 1932 the CDC's predecessor organization, the US PHS, had begun a study of untreated syphilis in African-American men in the city of Tuskegee, Alabama. Men were told they would receive special, free medical treatment if they would help the government learn about a "bad blood" disease. What the US PHS was actually doing was testing and identifying men with syphilis, then concealing the syphilis diagnosis from the infected men so that doctors could observe the progression of syphilis.

The scientific rationale for the Tuskegee Experiment's study design was that much was unknown about untreated syphilis' effects on the body, and that pre-penicillin syphilis treatments may have been doing more harm than good (e.g., arsenic was a common syphilis treatment at the time). The ethical "rationale" for concealing the syphilis diagnosis from poor black sharecropping men, and performing multiple invasive tests like spinal taps, was that poor black men in the South were unlikely to receive any treatment for syphilis anyway, and the findings from their sacrifice would benefit mankind.

None of those excuses would ever make sense to anyone with a rudimentary sense of morality. Still, the US PHS removed any justification for its actions in 1934 by publishing a paper detailing the ill effects of untreated syphilis on the body. Even worse, in 1943, three US Marine Hospital physicians discovered that penicillin completely cured syphilis when administered in the primary or secondary stage, but *not* after the infection progressed to latent or tertiary syphilis.

Those revelations should have immediately put a halt to the Tuskegee Experiment, thereby saving lives and lessening the suffering of the infected men and their families. Instead, there was a mere bureaucratic reshuffling: the US PHS quietly transferred its portfolio over to the new CDC, who let the project continue without any reassessment of its purpose or ethics.

By 1957, the entire US PHS Venereal Disease Division was officially the domain of the CDC. Since one of the Venereal Disease Division's tasks was to set up rapid treatment centers where intramuscular injections of penicillin were given to cure syphilis, the CDC had another prime opportunity to put a halt to the Tuskegee Experiment. At that time, as bureaucrats would say, the CDC had not "owned" the Tuskegee Experiment for any length of time, and so it could have shifted blame onto the disappearing US PHS. However, when the CDC arrived in Tuskegee to administer penicillin injections, curiously no one enrolled in the Tuskegee Experiment was treated. The opportunity to eradicate syphilis from hundreds of men – as well as prevent syphilis infection in their sexual partners and children – was lost.

Moreover, the CDC continued the Tuskegee Experiment for another fifteen years, following those men and their families until a whistleblower came forward in 1972. The total number of victims is unknown, although historians believe that perhaps over a hundred men likely died of untreated syphilis, at least 40 female partners contracted the disease, and at least 19 children were born with congenital syphilis.

It's little wonder that the blowback continues today. The African-American community rightly cites the Tuskegee Experiment as historical evidence of the US government public health machinery's malfeasance against vulnerable citizens.

Bringing up the CDC's lurid history inevitably leads to CDC advocates declaring, *"But polio! We beat polio!"* The CDC's employees and media lackeys continually imply that the CDC was behind the vaccination effort that eradicated endemic polio from the US. However, the real hero behind the polio eradication effort was the National Foundation for Infantile Paralysis (the precursor to today's March of Dimes Foundation). That private foundation in the 1950s used donations to organize a polio vaccine clinical trial with 1.8 million pediatric participants. To put that feat in perspective, the COVID-19 vaccine trials run by big pharma had around 40,000 participants each. Additionally, a vaccine trial organized by a non-government, non-academic organization would be nearly impossible today with the FDA's byzantine regulations.

The polio vaccine trial was successful, and soon thereafter the US began a mass vaccination campaign. However, there was an early setback when a bad batch of polio vaccine caused 250 cases of actual polio. What happened next could never have happened had the government been in charge. The National Foundation for Infantile Paralysis, being a mission-oriented organization aiming to improve society, went back to the drawing board with the vaccine scientists, and the bad batch problem was corrected. The vaccination campaign then resumed because the public trusted the National Foundation for Infantile Paralysis, since its original activity was using donations to pay for polio treatment for children whose families who could not afford it. Therefore, the polio vaccination campaign continued towards ultimate success, and the last known case of polio in the US occurred in 1979.

While the CDC's proponents would be correct in stating that the CDC is part of a worldwide global polio immunization program, that brings up the CDC's activities in foreign countries that don't directly or even indirectly benefit US citizens. Of the CDC's requested $6.6 billion budget in 2020, nearly half of that money went abroad ($2.6 billion to global efforts to fight tuberculosis, Ebola, and malaria, and $457 million to general global disease protection programs). We should be very skeptical of money sent abroad for CDC foreign activities given the CDC's history of choosing foreign partners.

Take the CDC's relationship with Saddam Hussein's Iraq as a prime example. While not well publicized, the CDC stores and studies deadly pathogens like smallpox, Ebola, and other potential biologic weapons at its Atlanta laboratories. Even less well publicized is that the CDC has sent some of those deadly substances to other countries. Between 1984 and 1989, the CDC sent strains of anthrax bacteria, botulinum toxin, and West Nile virus to the University of Baghdad. At the time, the US was friendly with Saddam Hussein's Iraq and was supporting Iraq against Iran in the Iran-Iraq War. However, the "enemy of my enemy is my friend" style of foreign diplomacy doesn't necessarily have to extend to sharing anthrax spores. As United Nations (UN) weapons inspector Jonathan Tucker later noted, "*...they [CDC] did deliver samples that Iraq said had a legitimate public health purpose, which I think was naïve to believe.*" According to the UN, the University of Baghdad was a front for Saddam's biological weapons program, and the CDC's samples were potentially the starter kit for biological weapons used by Iraq against Iran in the Iran-Iraq War.

Whether naïve or part of a covert US military initiative, certainly the CDC's shipments of biologic weapons to Iraq was stupid. However, lessons learned from that episode, if any were learned, would not dissuade the CDC from volunteering for future military misadventures. Post-9/11, the CDC's mission statement was updated to include national security language such as, "safety and security threats" and "health security." Stay tuned for future disasters when effete public health bureaucrats decide they want to run and gun with the Department of Defense and the CIA.

Back stateside, the CDC's missions are now less medical and more nanny state. While CDC originally stood for Communicable Disease Center, that was changed to Centers for Disease Control in 1970, and Prevention was added in 1992. The addition of Prevention officially extended the CDC's reach far beyond fighting infectious diseases to current "threats" such as tobacco smoke, obesity, chronic diseases, and workplace hazards (now to include brutish unvaccinated people trying to make a living).

With infectious diseases on the wane in America due to traditional childhood vaccines and antibiotics, the CDC pivoted to its Prevention mission in the 1990s. Savvy readers will note that government agencies always pivot after a series of misadventures. In the case of the CDC, the pivot came after the fallout from the Tuskegee Experiment revelations and shipments of anthrax to a murderous dictator. The public face of the pivot was broadening the CDC's mission to include healthcare issues that were historically the purview of the individual doctor-patient relationship. But behind closed doors, the CDC was also looking to secure its bloated annual budget just in case some eager, ambitious congressman started following the paper trail of CDC money leaving the US. Hence, the CDC Foundation was born.

Potentially a model upon which the Clinton Foundation was designed, the CDC Foundation is a private nonprofit organization which melds the CDC's governmental mission with private sector money. The CDC Foundation funds projects focused on random foreign problems that in no way could ever affect Americans – like "Improving Understanding of Drowning in Africa." Despite being a private entity, the CDC Foundation's creation was authorized by federal statute. And much like the Clinton Foundation, the CDC Foundation's board members and advisors are a Who's Who list of insurance, hospital, academic, and think tank strategists who need a cushy and well-compensated side job.

While the CDC Foundation funds hundreds of pet programs, the CDC proper has become obsessed with moralizing to Americans over issues such as smoking. While smoking could be left up to personal choice, individual responsibility, and private conversations between patient and doctor, the CDC wants Americans to know that smoking endangers us all (foreshadowing their COVID-19 vaccine messaging). And while the CDC cries that smoking is an activity that endangers everyone, the CDC also asserts that smoking is never the fault of the individual.

In fact, smoking is a by-product of systematic racism and discriminatory attitudes towards the transgender community. Yes, you read that right. The CDC is particularly concerned about the transgender population and their allies smoking, writing on their website that, *"Bartenders and servers in LGBT nightclubs are exposed to high levels of secondhand smoke."* Never mind that people smoke in all types of places, or perhaps that people smoke to relieve stress after the media says to prevent COVID-19 you must wear four face masks. Regardless, all of the CDC's preventative medical initiatives, including smoking, are an insincere power play. A particularly rich example of that insincerity was when former CDC Director Dr. Brenda Fitzgerald had to resign after it was revealed she bought shares in a tobacco company – while CDC Director.

The media historically has done a great job glossing over the CDC's true history, as it wasn't until the COVID-19 pandemic that the public began to realize that the CDC is not the world's greatest public health organization. Various polls show that Americans' trust in the CDC is falling. Government and academic acolytes emboldened by the Biden administration are rallying to try and turn that tide of souring public opinion. But don't be fooled. Real public health interests like banning carcinogenic pesticides and endocrine disrupting chemicals could be a powerful argument for the existence and authority of government public health agencies, but in practice those agencies are hardly ever effective and typically cause more harm than good.

Just as the CDC grew out of the post-WWII government baby boom, so too did the NIH. Before WWII, the US government started a National Cancer Institute. After WWII, that Institute became one of many institutes, and today the NIH is comprised of 27 very well-funded institutes and centers. From an initial budget of $4 million in 1947, Congress has exponentially grown the NIH's budget to nearly $42 billion in 2020. Despite the continual faux outrage from the media about decreased funding for medical research (e.g., blaming the 1980s HIV crisis on Republican spending cuts), the NIH's budget is the envy of most other government institutions, save the Pentagon.

What do Americans receive in return for their tax dollars? The NIH's budget supports biomedical research, both internal research at NIH's hospital and laboratories in Bethesda, Maryland, and external research at US academic universities (and apparently in Wuhan, China too). Internal research projects are guided by NIH leadership, with money allocated to the various institutes who hire research staff to spearhead those programs. But external research is the gravy train, with 80% of NIH funding allocated to outsourced science projects, in many cases with little to no oversight.

The COVID-19 pandemic put a harsh but overdue spotlight on how the NIH selects, funds, and regulates those external research projects. But to those with knowledge of how those "extramural" programs work, the grant word-smithing around gain-of-function research and the lax oversight of EcoHealth Alliance's activities at the Wuhan Institute of Virology was not surprising at all. To understand how taxpayer funded biomedical research potentially made a pandemic possible, let's follow the journey of an NIH extra-mural grant proposal.

Imagine you're a medical researcher who wants to study COVID-19 virus variants. In 2021, COVID-19 variants like Delta and Omicron exposed the existing COVID-19 vaccines as less effective than initially advertised. You and your laboratory want to create new COVID-19 variants and test vaccines on them. This is all in the name of preventing future problems, of course.

Your application to the NIH is due in 12 months. You spend the year leading up to the deadline traveling to conferences and wining and dining your colleagues. Meanwhile, your PhD students work long hours in the laboratory creating COVID-19 variants, funded by money from your previous grants.

You return from conferences well-fed, rested, and ready to write a grant proposal outlining: 1) the urgent need for your research, 2) the innovative ways your lab *will* create and study these variants (note future tense here), and 3) the future implications of your work – i.e., we can fix the COVID-19 vaccine trainwreck and save face for government and big pharma.

You submit your application to NIH. One might assume that it is NIH staff who review these external applications, but that is not what happens. NIH outsources the review of extramural applications by assembling "study sections," which are echo-chamber groups of academics who typically have received NIH funding. A group of colleagues who research COVID-19 (and maybe some who helped create COVID-19) will be judging your COVID-19 variant grant proposal. Fortunately for you, you just spent the last year wining and dining those very same colleagues at conferences.

Study section meetings last several days, during which time academic researchers take turns reviewing applications while boasting about their own past achievements. On paper, the meetings are an impartial review, debate, and scoring of grant applications. What happens in reality is that study section members are naturally more favorable to grant applications that validate their own studies. Compounding this is that study section members, having successfully been funded by NIH, are already a group that aligns their beliefs and interests to those of the NIH. Thus, the NIH controls the players and referees in the grants game. And since the NIH is the largest funder of biomedical research in the world, it therefore controls what research questions are asked and answered.

Back to your COVID-19 variant application – it receives a great score from the study section since you are proposing a solution not just to a medical problem, but a political problem as well. The study section scores are routed to an NIH committee which reviews the scores, selects the winning applications, and decides on how much money to award to each.

You receive a notice of award!

It is at this moment, rather late in the process, when the NIH's staff responsible for oversight and adherence to federal regulations look at your proposal for the first time. It seems as if you are proposing a project that could be construed as gain-of-function research (creating new COVID-19 variants that could be deadlier than existing variants). This is a sore subject for the NIH. The NIH oversight team emails you asking for clarification: *"Surely you will not intentionally make these variants deadly? Your lab protocols and security follow rigid standards? Of course, you will notify us if something bad happens, right?"* (A nearly identical exchange happened between NIH oversight staff and EcoHealth Alliance head Peter Daszak).

You reply, *"Yes, we do everything by the book in my lab,"* referencing your extensive safety record. Meanwhile, your PhD students have already created seven COVID-19 variants and you've got a manuscript ready to submit for peer-reviewed publication as soon as the timing won't raise suspicion. That is the secret to NIH grant success: have the work nearly done by the time you get the grant. Unfortunately, that secret was overlooked by the media in 2021 when a disturbing EcoHealth Alliance grant proposal that was not funded by the US government was made public. That unsuccessful grant proposal to the Department of Defense was for a gain-of-function research project creating extra-virulent coronaviruses. The media painted the revelation as a "near miss" story, but given Daszak's success with previous federal grants, this author's educated guess is that the project's gain-of-function aims had already been completed.

If the work funded by a new grant is already complete, then what do you do with the grant money? The answer is support your existing academic salary and hire more graduate students, so that you can start working on the next, more ambitious grant proposal, ensuring your grant funding will continue indefinitely. It also helps that once you're in the club of NIH-funded researchers, it is a self-sustaining, insular group. Despite their proclamations of diversity, the NIH is an old boys club, with the same group of mostly male, mostly white scientists repeatedly winning prestigious, multi-million-dollar R01 awards year after year.

You and your lab team wait a year after the grant starts, publish a preliminary data paper, and then wait another year before publishing a bigger, definitive paper. Meanwhile, you work on the next big idea (unexpected yet beneficial side effects of the sixth COVID-19 booster shot!). Your university employer is very happy with you since the NIH gives universities additional funds, in addition to your grant award money, called indirect costs. Indirect costs are like slush funds that universities get to spend indiscriminately. You are on the fast track to promotion and will likely get funding from the NIH again. And maybe now you will also be invited to be a member of an NIH study section.

Balancing its dysfunctional grants system are the important medical discoveries that were funded by the NIH. (Whether those discoveries present a net benefit to society is up for debate). That said, the NIH has had a Jekyll and Hyde history from its inception, with sordid scandals alternating with scientific breakthroughs. Indeed, the NIH's current level of dysfunction and dangerous research outsourced to China may not hold a candle to earlier misadventures.

At the same time that government was expanding into medicine during the post-WWII Cold War period, military and intelligence agencies were focusing their growing powers on combating communist enemies. The CIA's ARTICHOKE, BLUEBIRD, MK-NAOMI, and most notably, MK-ULTRA programs leveraged that power for sinister goals. Led by chemist Sidney Gottlieb, MK-ULTRA was an ultimately failed attempt to understand how lysergic acid diethylamide (LSD) and other psychedelics could be weaponized for use as mind control against communists (or against anyone the US government declared a threat). Although CIA henchmen traveled abroad to kidnap people for their most heinous experiments, they also ran experiments on US citizens stateside. Conveniently, the army provided Fort Detrick as a clandestine Maryland home base for Gottlieb and MK-ULTRA.

Despite the shield of Fort Detrick, the CIA and the military never want to be the front men. Therefore, many of MK-ULTRA's 149 known sub-projects were outsourced to the NIH and academic institutions via sham non-profit foundations and through real foundations such as the Rockefeller and Macy foundations. The stated aim of those projects was to help advance the treatment of addiction, depression, and other mental health problems. In reality, the CIA was paying academic researchers to recruit both regular and troubled Americans to be unwitting recipients of LSD and other mind-altering substances (including methamphetamines, mescaline, and psilocybin, among others), often given at astronomically high doses and for prolonged periods of time.

NIH's involvement was mainly through its National Institute of Mental Health (NIMH). NIMH performed studies for MK-ULTRA as well as awarded grants to academic institutions to further outsource MK-ULTRA work. Grant recipients included prestigious universities such as Harvard, Cornell, Princeton, and Yale, as well as more obscure institutions like Mendocino State Mental Hospital, which had ready access to vulnerable heroin addicts seeking treatment. Potentially creating the future Unabomber out of the shy but brilliant Harvard undergraduate Ted Kaczynski, and feeding the downward spiral of heroin addicts in California, the NIMH for decades aided and abetted in heinous and unethical experimentation upon innocent Americans.

The extent of the NIH's involvement and active collaboration with the CIA and Sidney Gottlieb is unknown, as public knowledge of MK-ULTRA is based upon the discovery in the 1970s of relatively few documents (Gottlieb and the CIA were notorious for lack of documentation and for destroying evidence). As detailed in the books *Poisoner in Chief* by Stephen Kinzer and *A Terrible Mistake* by H.P. Albarelli Jr., the poor Americans driven insane or to suicide by LSD and other MK-ULTRA experiments are likely only part of the entire horror story.

Today the NIH has still not shed its habit of funding unethical experimentation. Aside from the EcoHealth Alliance's work at the Wuhan Institute of Virology, another recent scandal involves a $3 million NIMH grant to a child psychiatrist at University of Illinois at Chicago. Those grant funds were used for the administration of the psychotropic drug lithium to children younger than the authorized age. Although the NIMH's internal review casts blame entirely on

University of Illinois' research regulators, study issues were reported to NIMH several times before any action was taken to protect children too young to give informed consent.

As of this writing, the NIH is currently funding a study, perversely named MyPEEPS, that pays minors hundreds of dollars to report their sexual activity on a smart phone app. Because those minors are too young to legally consent for participation in a research study, both the NIH and the principal investigator's employer Columbia University decided that the study could proceed with a waiver of informed consent. Never mind the potential for breach of data privacy when sexual details are shared on a smart phone app, never mind that parents have a right to know when their child is in a research study, and never mind that several hundred dollars compensation is quite coercive in getting a teenager to reveal their sexual activity – somehow this study will help "prevent HIV."

How will the public know if MyPEEPS actually prevents HIV? In many cases, the results of NIH-funded research are hard to find outside of academic journals that can only be read by paying subscribers. Yet by law NIH-funded research is supposed to be reported to the public website ClinicalTrials.gov. However, a STAT investigation found that many researchers fail to report or fail to make a timely report of their study results to ClinicalTrials.gov.

The NIH is supposed to use tax dollars to fund research that benefits US citizens. But just as the CDC uses the CDC

Foundation, the NIH uses the John Edward Fogarty International Center to send US taxpayer money overseas. The Fogarty Center not only funds US researchers working abroad on global health projects, but it also funds foreign researchers working in their own country on projects unrelated to the US. Representative examples of Fogarty-funded projects include research on Alzheimer's disease in rural Colombia and establishing a bioethics training program in India.

Though its annual budget of $54 million is relatively small, the Fogarty Center has funded thousands of projects since 1968. In their own words, Fogarty is the *"bridge between NIH and the greater global health community."* Except Fogarty means the greater global health community that the US State Department designates as America-friendly. Under the pretense of supporting "low- and middle-income countries," in 2012 the NIH announced that China, Russia, Turkey, and other Russia-friendly Baltic states were ineligible for Fogarty grants. Thus, Fogarty grants, like many other items in the federal budget, are essentially bribes and handouts to members of the US State Department clique.

Fogarty's exclusion of Chinese researchers is particularly amusing, as the NIH has been unwittingly sending money, intellectual property, and trained biomedical researchers to China for decades. In 2018, the US Senate Committee on Homeland Security and Governmental Affairs began investigating the NIH's inadvertent role in building up China's biomedical capabilities. The committee's report details the NIH's lax compliance efforts in ensuring research and intellectual property were kept stateside. Researchers receiving NIH grants are bound by law to disclose if they are engaged in any foreign activities, receive any foreign or industry money, or otherwise have any other conflicts of interest. The US Senate report revealed that the NIH did not verify researcher disclosures, but instead followed an honors system. One NIH staffer admitted the vetting process for researchers' potential conflicts of interest was limited to reviewing the first page of internet search results for the researcher's name.

Taking advantage of the US government being sound asleep at the wheel, China has sent academic researchers to America to apply for and receive NIH grants for decades, and it has recruited Chinese nationals and US citizens who already had NIH funding for their Thousand Talents Program. What ensued was cash payments from the Chinese government to NIH-funded researchers, in exchange for sending confidential research discoveries and intellectual property to China. In more extreme cases, Thousand Talents Program participants were paid to set up laboratories in China to work in parallel with their NIH-funded efforts in the US, essentially copying and pasting the US-funded research playbook.

The Thousand Talents Program was (and perhaps still is) massive in scope. A Department of Justice investigation identified nearly 400 suspected participants with NIH and other government funding at some of the most prestigious academic medical institutions in the US (including Harvard,

MD Anderson Cancer Center, and University of California, to name a few). Although investigations are still ongoing, universities have been fined millions of dollars for improper grants management, and some researchers have been jailed over their failure to disclose significant financial relationships with China (e.g., Charles Lieber, the former head of Harvard's chemistry department).

Although universities with billion-dollar endowments involved in the Thousand Talents scandal may be fined millions of dollars, the NIH will not suffer at all for its lack of oversight. In fact, each individual NIH institute functions as its own fiefdom with little to no consequences for failure or missteps.

The most prescient example of that is Dr. Anthony Fauci, long the head of the National Institute of Allergy and Infectious Diseases (NIAID). Even before COVID-19, Fauci repeatedly failed forward to become the highest paid of all federal government employees. Responding to HIV in the 1980s and to the post-9/11 anthrax attacks, Fauci redirected NIAID's budget towards completely unsuccessful efforts to develop HIV and anthrax vaccines (story sound familiar?). Despite billions of dollars spent, today there is no widely accepted HIV or anthrax vaccine, although the US military forced an anthrax vaccine on its soldiers and those who refused were discharged or harshly punished (again, sound familiar?).

Much described here about the CDC and NIH also extends to other health-related government agencies, like the National Science Foundation (NSF). Readers of former US Senator Tom Coburn's annual list of government waste may recall the NSF's funding of a $3 million grant studying how shrimp run on treadmills underwater.

Another medical research agency you might have never heard of with a massive budget is the Patient-Centered Outcomes Research Institute (PCORI). PCORI was created by the Affordable Care Act, operates with annual budgets north of $2 billion, and is run by a board of directors that reports to no one. PCORI's projects read like a well-funded struggle session: $6.8 million for "Leveraging mHealth and Peers to Engage African-Americans and Latinxs in HIV Care," and $1.4 million for "Peer online motivational interviewing for sexual and gender minority male survivors."

Then there is the interesting Agency for Healthcare Research and Quality (AHRQ). AHRQ's budget is relatively paltry ($436 million in 2021), yet its stated interests are areas that should receive the most funding (e.g., decreasing diagnostic errors and fighting antibiotic-resistant bacteria). Yet in medical research circles it is well known that AHRQ is the poor, ugly stepchild attempting to do actual work. Researchers are often discouraged from applying for AHRQ grants. Odds of funding are better if one applies to NSF or PCORI for funding to study if watching shrimp run on treadmills underwater alleviates depression in HIV-positive Latinos.

Just as nearly every government agency became involved in the anti-terror mission after 9/11, government agencies have schemed for years on how to benefit (i.e., increase funding and job security) from a pandemic. While the NIH was funding gain-of-function research that may have caused the COVID-19 pandemic, federal government bureaucrats from both Republican and Democrat administrations were planning exactly how to expand their powers in the event of a medical crisis.

Those schemes are outlined in the "Pandemic Playbook," a document reportedly passed down through multiples presidential administrations that details how the federal government should respond to *"high-consequence emerging infectious disease threats and biological incidents."* Early in the COVID-19 pandemic, Politico published the playbook, likely in attempt to show that the Trump administration was failing to follow its instructions on how to save Americans. Assuming that document is authentic, the reality was that government agencies, to the extent they could under Trump, were following the Playbook step-by-step.

Now under the Biden administration we are seeing the more Orwellian suggestions from the Playbook come to life. Section II, entitled "Exercising the Playbook," calls for the coordination and meetings of, *"at a minimum...representatives from HHS (including the CDC, NIH, ASPR, OGA, and others), DOL/OSHA, DOD, DOT, USAID, DOS, DHS, USDA, EPA, and members of the Intelligence Community."*

Savvy readers will recognize this call for coordination between government agencies as exactly what happened post-9/11. And just as the post-9/11 security state led to widespread curtailing of freedoms, the post-COVID-19 security state has led to censoring of speech, barring citizens from working and participating in commerce, the purging of military and healthcare professionals, and databases tracking those who have not received a COVID-19 vaccination.

Amidst the creepy Orwellian phrases and calls for expansion of the national spy state, the Playbook is filled with bureaucratic jargon and run-on sentences seemingly devoid of verbs, least of all actual actionable recommendations. In fact, 16 of its 69 pages merely list different agencies and councils that need to be included in any US pandemic response. But nowhere in the Playbook are historical insights from past pandemics. It took decades before doctors figured out the 1918 pandemic was a virus. Back then, many scientists initially thought that the influenza viral pandemic was caused by a bacterium. More recently, HIV was initially thought to be a cancer, and its mechanism of transmission was unknown for years. Yet at every step during the COVID-19 pandemic, the US government has acted as though its knowledge of the virus was complete and absolute.

Put simply, the US government role in healthcare is a woeful combination of "big Army stupid" and third-world inefficient. So long as the media help cover up or set in a memory hole government mistakes, and bureaucrats check all their boxes, there is no danger to the existence or expansion of government healthcare agencies (which now spend $1 out of every $4 dollars in the federal budget). The reality is that a government bureaucrat's survival relies on creating more problems, even if those are health problems that endanger the survival of citizens.

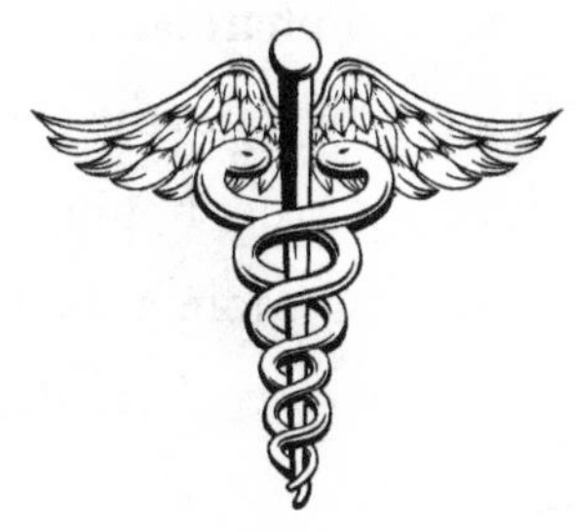

BIG PHARMA & THE FDA: REGULATORY CAPTURE

"Disease is the biggest money maker in our economy."

—John H. Tobe

"If you have a drug that is $100 for one course of therapy, and you know that you can charge $100,000, what should shareholders think when you say, 'I'd rather not take the heat'?"

—Martin Shkreli

While the media distracts Americans with a false debate on the future of American healthcare between government-planned socialism versus free market capitalism, the unspoken third option is unopposed and going strong. That third option, our current reality, is an alliance between government and corporations.

However, in the realm of pharmaceutical drugs, terming this partnership an alliance overstates the government's power in the relationship. "Junior partner hoping to be useful so he doesn't get fired," would be a more accurate description of the power dynamics in this case of regulatory capture. It's the well-functioning pharmaceutical corporations that call the shots and reap the profits, and big pharma likely views government and the Food and Drug Administration (FDA) as "the corpse to which we are chained."

Yet at the same time, it is true that pharmaceutical corporations could not have grown into the behemoths they are today, exerting oligarchical power, without government backing. The FDA approves big pharma's products and federal laws allow pharmaceutical companies to avoid liability for products like vaccines.

The government also permissively allows pharma to buy off doctors – about half of physicians receive payments from industry. Contrary to doctors' protestations, those payments do influence prescriptions for everything from opioids to diabetes drugs. Left out of consideration are those who pay for the drugs and put them into their bodies: the patients.

Prior to the 2020 presidential election, a poll reported that three-quarters of Americans surveyed said the cost of prescription medicines would influence their vote. In the midst of the Trump-Russiagate fervor, both political parties were oblivious to the fact that the average American was spending $1,229 per year on prescription and over-the-counter drugs.

Drug prices had steadily increased while the 2008 and 2020 economic crisis left the majority of Americans with less than $1,000 in savings.

Cue the chorus of normie conservative editorials: *"But the free market! That's the price of research and development (R&D)! If pharmaceutical companies can't charge a fair market price, we'll be like Cuba and Venezuela!"*

But big pharma does not operate in a free market, because there is enormous asymmetry of information with regards to the efficacy of their products. The other truth is that pharmaceutical companies do not pay the full price of R&D. Yet R&D is the reflexive corporatist defense against inflated drug prices, pharma executive bonuses, and amoral, excessive profiting off disease and suffering.

Pharmaceutical companies want you to believe that they alone spend astronomical amounts bringing a drug to market (i.e., the journey from a molecule in a test tube to a pill at your local pharmacy). So just how much does R&D cost? Median drug development costs are between $648-$985 million. The potential payoff for that investment is a median total revenue of $1.66 billion. Making pharmaceutical drugs therefore seems high-risk, high reward.

Except big pharma has figured out how to decrease that financial risk. It turns out that many of the costs of drug development are born by the US government, either in the form of direct taxpayer subsidies (as was the case during Operation Warp Speed for COVID-19 vaccines), or in the outsourcing of drug development tasks to the NIH and academic institutions. At the end of the day, Americans end up paying twice for their drugs – first with their tax dollars and second at the pharmacy. To understand how that happens, and how big pharma obfuscates the results of drug trials, let's follow a drug through all phases of development.

Drug development has come a long way from the methods by which Alexander Fleming isolated penicillin, the first antibiotic, from mold. Scientists at pharmaceutical companies used to painstakingly isolate and manually test hundreds or even thousands of molecules for their potential as therapeutic drugs. Now, in the age of machine learning, initial drug development and testing are largely performed by supercomputers running algorithms and repeated simulations. Supercomputer-powered drug development is relatively inexpensive and increases the likelihood of finding a promising molecule and in doing so in less time.

Of note, this "exploratory phase" is not always conducted in-house at pharmaceutical companies. Conveniently for big pharma, the NIH spends over 50% of its budget searching for promising molecules and trying to better understand how diseases impair bodily function at the cellular level. How often does that taxpayer-funded basic science research at the NIH assist big pharma? Nearly all of time. The FDA approved 210 new molecular entities between 2010-2016, and NIH studies either identified or contributed to work on every single one of those molecules.

After promising molecules are identified, those molecules are tested in laboratory experiments using isolated human cells (sometimes cells from aborted fetuses). Following success in isolated cells, the first round of testing in animals begins, but this also can be outsourced to the NIH or to universities. Animals are selected for their relevant anatomic or physiologic similarity to humans. For example, rhesus macaque monkeys are often used to test vaccines, including vaccines for the original SARS virus and recently vaccines for COVID-19. (Of note, the original SARS vaccine trials did not end well for the monkeys, with antibody-dependent enhancement causing horrible lung disease and death. Hence, there is no original SARS vaccine, and this is one of the many reasons why some doctors, including this author, are hesitant to take a COVID-19 vaccine.) Assuming the animals don't die during this first round of live testing, they are killed and dissected to see whether the experimental drug was helpful or harmful.

If testing goes well with animals, then it becomes time to involve real humans and the FDA. Pharmaceutical companies submit an Investigational Drug Application (IND) to the FDA asking to proceed with human clinical trials. That IND application contains information from the exploratory phase and animal testing, but typically is also synchronized with lobbyist activity and media stories hinting at a new breakthrough drug. Once the IND is approved by the FDA, the three phases of clinical trials can begin.

Understanding the FDA-required phases of clinical trials is crucial to evaluating a new drug and its potential efficacy. A lack of understanding of that process is why breathless media pronouncements about "game-changer" COVID-19 therapeutic drugs and vaccines, which went a great way to keeping the stock market soaring, were wholly irresponsible.

Additionally, media coverage of those studies implied that they were being conducted by the pharmaceutical companies themselves. Yet over the last decade the NIH has itself performed more and more of those Phase 1-3 clinical trials on behalf of the pharmaceutical industry. Big pharma supplies the pills and some money, and the NIH puts out notices to universities and academic hospitals that they need help running a drug trial, and thus the actual trial is doubly outsourced. Universities and hospitals sign up to be sites for the trial, hire a study team using a mix of pharmaceutical and NIH/taxpayer money, give the drug to patients following a study protocol written by the pharmaceutical company, and deal with any real human complications.

In Phase 1 of this process, the drug is tested in a small number of healthy young people (usually between 10 - 50 people). The reason for testing a drug first in a small number of healthy volunteers is to see if there are any catastrophic side effects, and so by design the dose tested in Phase 1 is very small. If the first few volunteers don't get sick, the dose is gradually increased until either the drug company feels that it is a sufficient therapeutic dose, or until the participants begin to experience adverse effects. The average length of a Phase 1 trial is 15 months. Compare that with the timeline of Operation Warp Speed, which blasted through Phases 1 - 3 in less than 12 months.

Assuming there are no atrocious side effects or deaths during Phase 1, the drug company will ask the FDA for permission to proceed to Phase 2, and about 70% of drugs move on from Phase 1 to Phase 2. While a stock market analyst might think that sounds like a great statistic for next quarter's earnings report, it also means that nearly one-third of Phase 1 drugs had serious or intolerable side effects in healthy young volunteers.

In Phase 2, a few hundred people with the disease of interest are given the drug to monitor for side effects, to test different doses, and begin to measure whether the drug treats the disease in question. As with Phase 1, the average Phase 2 trial lasts 16 months; however, only a third of drugs move on from Phase 2 to Phase 3. Unsurprisingly, when a drug is given to sicker, older people rather than healthy, younger people, there are going to be more side effects. Additionally, now that the drug's efficacy against disease is being tested, the drug may simply not work as intended.

If a drug makes it out of Phase 2 and into Phase 3, thousands of participants are randomly given either the new drug or a placebo (or, depending on the circumstances, to standard of care therapy). The goal of Phase 3 is to see whether the new drug is statistically superior to the placebo or standard of care. That takes time, and the average length of a Phase 3 trial is 17 months, although some Phase 3 trials take years. According to the FDA, only 25-30% of drugs make it out of Phase 3 to apply for actual FDA approval.

As you can imagine, at this stage in the process big pharma is now heavily invested in the drug's success and will pull out all the stops for a final FDA approval to bring the drug to market. So while big pharma outsources the messy business of dealing with patients in drug trials, it is big pharma's in-house statisticians who analyze the trial data. And those statisticians have crafty, ever-changing ways of performing statistical analyses so that the results nearly always support the drug's efficacy.

Randomly assigning participants into two groups and comparing their outcomes seems simple on paper, but statisticians can make it much more complicated. In "intent to treat analysis," data from a participant who dropped out of the trial can be used to favorably support the drug's efficacy. Never mind that the participant dropped out due to intolerable side effects, if the drug seemed to be working in that patient, their data will be included in the analysis. "Pragmatic" trial designs allow inclusion of data from people who forget to take the drug for days or even weeks, which may make a drug seem to have less frequent or fewer side effects. "Crossover" trial designs have participants who begin the trial taking the investigational drug eventually switch over to the placebo, and vice-versa. The crossover design supposedly enhances statistical rigor. However, depending on the length of time a drug needs to take effect, and the length of time it takes for side effects to appear, the crossover design may obscure the truth about a drug's efficacy as well as its side effects.

During the pandemic big pharma statisticians got especially creative, particularly in the case of Remdesivir, a drug for hospitalized COVID-19 patients. Remdesivir was tested with an "adaptive" study design, where a cocktail of other drugs were added to the drug trial. Such study designs are labeled as "pragmatic, real-world" trials, but adding other drugs into the mix confounds the evaluation of the new, experimental drug.

Big pharma statisticians will argue that some complex Bayesian theorem supports their methods. But common sense alone dictates that those study designs are flawed. Remember that the next time you hear news reports about promising study results from a drug trial.

Beyond creative statistical analyses, the fact that big pharma and not an independent group analyzes drug trial data has resulted in numerous declarations of highly effective drugs that were, in fact, not effective at all. Between 2000 - 2011, 102 drug trials were retracted, 73 for scientific misconduct and 29 for statistical or other reporting errors. Even in smaller drug trials done by seemingly independent research teams, it is a good bet that the researcher in charge has received industry money.

The practice of sending data to big pharma for covert statistical analysis runs in stark contrast to the open-source movement, which is starting to spread from computer science over to medicine. Some medical researchers are now stripping out information identifying their subjects and then voluntarily sharing their data so their studies can be replicated, yet only 25% of pharmaceutical companies are sharing any kind of data. In a functional system, US citizens and independent scientists would have access to de-identified data from all vaccine and drug trials. We paid for it, after all.

After Phase 3, companies can apply for FDA approval to bring the drug to market. If they are successful and the FDA approves the drug, the pharmaceutical company can begin marketing and selling their new product. Yet there is still one more Phase that is often overlooked. Phase 4 is also known as Post-Market Safety Monitoring and is supposed to identify long-term side effects and more rare side effects that appear only when the drug is given to a much larger population. But as we see with COVID-19 vaccines, Phase 4 is a joke. It is rare that pharmaceutical companies or the FDA will admit a mistake and backtrack on a drug that is already approved, even in the face of serious side effects such as myocarditis in young children.

The COVID-19 fiasco has only increased the subservient role of the NIH to big pharma in performing drug trials. From Remdesivir to COVID-19 vaccines, all were tested in humans with NIH money and NIH logistical coordination.

Because the government had promised billions of dollars to pharmaceutical companies for their final products before any trials had been conducted, there was enormous pressure for those running the trials to exclude unfavorable data like bad side effects, as we saw with whistleblower allegations from Pfizer's COVID-19 vaccine trial.

In addition to cherry-picking results for new drugs and vaccines, big pharma also works in concert with government to disparage alternative drugs as ineffective. Case in point: before Trump made the drug hydroxychloroquine a political issue, that drug was doomed from the start. Why? Because it's a generic and costs a few dollars per pill. So hydroxychloroquine underwent a political and academic smear campaign, including publication of a study that convinced untold numbers of credulous doctors that not only was hydroxychloroquine ineffective in treating COVID-19, but it was dangerous. Although that study was eventually retracted, the damage was done: doctors educated to comply rather than think critically continue to disparage hydroxychloroquine (as well as the similarly smeared ivermectin) as an ineffective COVID-19 treatment.

By contrast, Remdesivir had potential for big profits. Thus, when analyzing Remdesivir's trial data, statisticians made the primary outcome the number of days people were sick instead of the outcome of greatest interest, death. Since a patient can only be included in the sick day analysis if he hasn't died, the results looked great because they contained only the subset of patients who ultimately lived. The exclusion of patients who died may have masked an important concern by many doctors, including myself, that Remdesivir caused organ failure and actually *increased* mortality.

As COVID-19 vaccines became available worldwide, the public began to see the disconnect between big pharma-controlled drug trials and what happens in real life, as well as the effects of the accelerated Operation Warp Speed timeline for COVID-19 vaccine testing. The astronomically high efficacy rates reported in Phase 3 trials for the Pfizer, Moderna, and Johnson & Johnson vaccines now appear to approach zero well within a year's time (a result that would have been revealed by the length of a traditional Phase 3 trial). And just as with Remdesivir, the COVID-19 vaccine trial outcomes were not "prevents COVID-19 infection," but rather "prevents severe COVID-19 infection."

While the phases of testing a new drug were originally designed with rigor and reproducibility in mind, today the entire FDA drug approval process is akin to Kabuki theatre. The dirty work of running the drug trials is outsourced to the NIH and academic institutions. Imaginative statisticians at pharmaceutical companies dream up new outcomes and statistical methods that will generate results that please their bosses. Those at the FDA don't live in a bubble – they want to put out press releases that send the stock market soaring and with it, their 401k and future prospects of a job at a pharmaceutical company. Drugs are approved for mass distribution, and then pharma, the FDA, and the NIH turn a blind eye to the real-world consequences.

Is big pharma satisfied with blockbuster new drugs developed with the help of the government? No, they are also busy devising ways to increase their revenues by extending patents and finding ways to make generics more expensive.

Patents give drug companies exclusive rights to produce and sell a new drug (i.e., a monopoly). When a patent expires the drug becomes generic, meaning any company can make and sell that drug. A typical drug patent lasts for 20 years, but the clock starts ticking when the drug is first invented. Given a typical (i.e., non-COVID-19) drug development timeline of 10 years, a drug company gets a decade or so of monopolistic selling and profiting off any drug that is *new and unique*. The definitions of "new" and "unique" are key to how drug companies extend patent protections beyond the 20-year timeline.

Insulin is a prime example of how big pharma gets creative extending patents. Insulin has been administered as a drug for diabetes since the 1920s. Although insulin was originally extracted from pigs, diabetics today inject synthetic human insulin made in laboratories. In addition to making a better, human insulin product, drug companies have also devised better ways to deliver the insulin. Instead of heroin chic syringes, insulin now comes in regular looking injectable pens with pre-filled doses – a new delivery mechanism that gives drug makers a new patent.

Diabetics worldwide have benefitted from those innovations, and until recently drug companies were honest brokers in setting prices for new insulin products. The original patent for insulin was sold for $1 by its altruistic Canadian discoverers. Eli Lilly's Humalog, a type of fast-acting insulin, cost $21 a vial in 1996. However, by 2019, that same Humalog delivered in an injectable pen cost $250 a vial. At a 2019 US Congressional hearing, an endocrinologist testified that insulin cost seven times more than it did twenty years ago, and as a result, many diabetics were rationing insulin (especially Type I diabetics, whose bodies do not make insulin and so rely on exogenous insulin to survive).

Insulin is not the only life-saving drug where big pharma's pricing preys upon people's fear of a premature death. Like insulin pens, EpiPens deliver a fixed amount of adrenaline to people experiencing a life-threatening allergic reaction known as anaphylaxis (e.g., after exposure to peanuts, shellfish, or a bee sting). Adrenaline has been used in medicine for over a hundred years, and thus has long been a generic drug. However, the EpiPen delivery mechanism is new and thus ripe for exploitation.

In 2007, a US pharmaceutical company called Mylan acquired the rights to manufacture and sell EpiPens. Again, because the active ingredient is generic, Mylan's rights didn't cover the drug itself, but rather the unique package of two EpiPens. Before Mylan's acquisition a package with two EpiPens cost about $100. After a decade of control by Mylan, the EpiPen package cost over $600, reaping annual sales of $1 billion for Mylan.

Public outcry ensued, especially since anaphylaxis is particularly life-threatening for young children. Corporate-friendly Republicans found themselves in an uncomfortable situation. While naturally oriented toward defending capitalist profiteering, Mylan's CEO was Heather Bresch, the daughter of Democrat Senator Joe Manchin. Indeed, that family connection had been key to Mylan's lobbying activities after they acquired the rights to EpiPen. Under the guise of community advocacy, Mylan successfully lobbied for state laws which made EpiPens mandatory in schools and other public places. Those bills passed while Mylan was jacking up the price of EpiPens by 500%. Mylan also allegedly gave money to pharmacy benefit managers in exchange for placing EpiPens on pharmacies' preferred list of drugs that are recommend to customers.

Congressional hearings ensued but were tempered by Republican and Democrat representatives who receive generous donations from drug companies. Mylan's concession was to reduce the price of the EpiPen package from $600 to $300, which got politicians great press for "taking on big pharma." Lost in the news coverage of this resolution was that the estimated price of manufacturing the EpiPen package was $10.

Insulin and EpiPens are just two of many examples of big pharma finding a lifesaving or life-sustaining drug, cornering the market using political lobbying and regulatory machinations, jacking up the price, and then counting the profits as they roll in. That formulaic and successful approach has been deployed for Hepatitis C treatment (Gilead's $1,000 pill), cancer therapies, new drugs for autoimmune diseases, COVID-19 therapeutics, "Pharma Bro" Martin Shkreli's anti-parasite drug, and many more.

And yet there are even more ways for big pharma to game the system, like drug expiration dates – largely inaccurate. For many drugs, more important than the arbitrary expiration date is the temperature at which drugs are stored. Another profit-increasing tactic is selecting two generic medications that are often taken together (e.g., two high blood pressure medications, or a pain reliever and a heartburn drug, or two HIV medications), and combining them into one pill. While the generic medications separately cost mere pennies, the one pill combination is "new and unique" and can be sold for exponentially more. It's the equivalent of combining $1 peanut butter and $2 chocolate and selling it as a Reese's candy for $500.

Exactly how much money does big pharma make using those tactics? Circa 2016, US citizens spent $480 billion on pharmaceutical drugs. Big pharma has friends and middlemen to pay off, and that year $73 billion went to pharmacies, $18 billion to drug wholesalers, $23 billion to pharmacy benefit managers, $35 billion to doctors, and $9 billion to insurers. But even after all those payoffs, there is still room for sky high profits. For example, before the COVID-19 vaccine, which is on par to be the biggest blockbuster drug of all time, Pfizer's annual gross profits were between $30 - $40 billion. Put another way, pharmaceutical companies' profit margins are on par with Wall Street's biggest, most profitable banks.

The political class in the US does a masterful job of protecting big pharma's status quo when inevitable public outrage ensues upon hearing of those profits. Republicans use scare-mongering tactics that claim any reform will instantly lead to socialism, and we'll be out of drugs like Cuba and Venezuela (conveniently forgetting the current major drug shortages in the US). Democrats propose regulations that would solidify the monopolistic authority of the biggest pharmaceutical companies and stifle competition from smaller competitors. And when Donald Trump as president expressed interest in lowering drug prices, the media portrayed fighting for lower prices as a "reckless attack" on hardworking companies.

Despite that propaganda, occasionally a sacrificial lamb is offered to stave off a French Revolution-style revolt. Most recently that was Purdue Pharma, the company that developed, manufactured, and sold OxyContin. Although many drug companies sold opioids and profited off a nation-wide opioid epidemic, the opioid crisis had become too big to ignore. Purdue Pharma's egregious marketing practices and kickbacks to "pill mill" doctors made them the perfect foil. Run privately by the privileged and tone-deaf Sackler family, aside from embarrassing universities and art museums endowed with their opioid riches, there was no threat to the stock market from the sacking of the Sacklers. Despite initial pushback from the Department of Justice, Purdue Pharma was eventually prosecuted and pled guilty to criminal charges. After fines totaling $4.5 billion, the company was dissolved. However, considering the greater than $13 billion in profits the Sackler family made from Oxycontin alone, one can debate the extent of their sacrifice.

Meanwhile, other drug companies continue to manufacture and market opioids at increasingly higher concentrations and win easy approval from friends at the FDA. Recently the FDA has approved two new ultrapotent opioids, Oliceridine and Sufentanil. Oliceridine is an intravenous opioid that is not needed at all considering hospitals already have morphine, fentanyl, and hydromorphone. Sufentanil is extremely dangerous as it is a tablet which dissolves under the tongue that produces a rapid and powerful high, and is meant for home use.

Sufentanil is so powerful that the chair of the FDA's Anesthetic and Analgesic Drug Products Advisory Committee urged the FDA to not even vote on its approval. Yet that FDA committee ultimately voted 10-3 in favor of Sufentanil's approval. While pill mills are shut down only to pop back up, and opioids destroy lives everywhere from Appalachia to inner cities, the FDA continues to stamp its seal of approval on newer and more addictive opioids, while the media distracts the public with stories of Purdue Pharma's downfall.

Unlike the CDC, NIH, and other government agencies which gained strength after WWII, the FDA's roots trace back further: to the late 19th and early 20th century Progressive political movement. Revelations about poor working conditions in the food industry detailed in *The Jungle* by Upton Sinclair gave progressives momentum, and subsequently several laws were passed regulating the food industry.

Food and pharmaceuticals were lumped together in 1906 when President Theodore Roosevelt signed the Pure Food and Drugs Act, which banned foreign and interstate traffic in "adulterated" or "misbranded" food, drugs, and liquor products. The law mandated that drug labels list active ingredients, although spared from disclosure were the preservatives and chemicals used to package drugs in pill or liquid form. The law also required the establishment of a National Formulary defining what constitutes a drug and standards for drug purity. Progressive and puritanical at the same time, the Pure Food and Drug Act's subsequent Sherley Amendments established the precursors of today's "Schedule" drugs (i.e., illegal drugs) by labeling the following addictive and dangerous: alcohol, morphine, opium, heroin, and cannabis indica (apparently Congress was unaware of the other type of marijuana, cannabis sativa).

The Pure Food and Drugs Act was ultimately stymied by its broad reach, as the government's attempt at its implementation and enforcement failed over the next twenty years. Thus, that law was replaced in 1938 with the Federal Food, Drug, and Cosmetic Act, signed by President Franklin Delano Roosevelt, who never missed an opportunity to increase the federal government's power. The Federal Food, Drug, and Cosmetic Act established the FDA and its control over food, drugs, medical devices, and cosmetics. Over the years the FDA has grown into a behemoth that regulates over $1 trillion of products annually, with authority over everything from cereal to condoms to COVID-19 vaccines.

If anyone questions why the FDA should have so much power, inevitably the scary story of thalidomide will be brought forth as *the* reason for the FDA. Thalidomide was a drug once prescribed in Europe to alleviate morning sickness in pregnant women. In the 1960s, when the FDA reviewed thalidomide for potential use in the US, there were already reports and pictures of European babies with horrendous birth defects born to mothers who had taken thalidomide. The FDA inspector assigned to thalidomide, Dr. Frances Kelsey, stalled the approval and asked for studies proving that thalidomide did not affect developing fetuses. Despite pressure from the pharmaceutical industry and her bosses at the FDA, Dr. Kelsey prevailed in blocking thalidomide's US approval. Thus, one of the FDA's greatest achievements was a doctor using common sense and resisting pressure from her bosses at the FDA.

But in the long history of the FDA, the thalidomide success story does not come close to balancing the harms the FDA has perpetrated against the American people.

The drug class called statins perfectly illustrates how big pharma always gets what it wants, how big pharma is aided at every step by the FDA, and how hapless doctors practice medicine without second guessing what they're told. Statins are widely prescribed drugs that lower blood cholesterol levels; in fact, one in four Americans over the age of 45 is taking a statin. That statistic reflects our obesity epidemic and the prescription-happy patterns of doctors. Reflecting greater societal issues, the thinking on both sides of a statin prescription is: Why would you stop eating junk or start lifting weights when you can just pop a pill? And those statin pills generate billions of dollars in profits for big pharma.

"That's money well-earned preventing heart attacks!" the normie conservative editorials will interject. There must be a reason for statins, right? And since they are prescribed to so many people, surely statins are safe? Before addressing safety, it's important to understand the purported reason why statins are prescribed, and why drug companies continue to invent new brand name statins.

What physicians are taught and then regurgitate to patients is that statins lower blood cholesterol levels. Because some studies show an association between high blood cholesterol levels and cardiovascular disease (emphasis on association and not proven causation), statins should theoretically reduce the risk of having a heart attack or stroke.

The first part of that premise is correct – statins will lower blood cholesterol levels. But as a good doctor would ask, does "treating the number" prevent disease? The answer is no. In a powerful type of study called a meta-analysis, data was pooled from 18 different randomized controlled trials and researchers found that to prevent 18 people from having a stroke or a heart attack, 1,000 people each had to take a statin for 5 consecutive years. Not exactly the powerful prevention you hear about in statins advertisements and from doctors.

And what was the response to that study from doctors and the medical establishment? *"We can prevent 18 people from having a heart attack!"* Yet to anyone with common sense, a success rate of 18 out of 1,000 people over a 5-year period seems rather ineffective. Regardless, the medical establishment has gone all-in on statins (remember the $35 billion big pharma pays to doctors every year), and statins are continually promoted in medical guidelines. Five of the ten steps of the American College of Cardiology's Guideline on the Management of Blood Cholesterol advise initiating a statin. Further reinforcing the need to use this cholesterol guideline is that the normal range for cholesterol keeps getting revised downward – a surefire way to guarantee that doctors write more statin prescriptions, and more patients take statins.

The love affair with statins would merely be an exercise in futility if it weren't for the fact that statins can be quite harmful. Aside from common drug side effects like allergic reactions and stomach issues, there are serious, even life-threatening statin side effects. The ideal patient would take a statin and begin exercising vigorously to lose weight and get healthy. Except statins can cause a condition called rhabdomyolysis, where in response to exercise (or simply to nothing at all) muscles break down and shed protein into the blood. The kidneys then attempt to filter the protein and are damaged, potentially irreversibly. That's what statins do to the big muscles of the body, but they also have been linked to weakening of the most important muscle, the heart.

As if causing heart problems while trying to prevent heart attacks wasn't counterproductive enough, statins also increase the risk of developing Type II diabetes. Many people being prescribed statins are already at-risk for developing Type II diabetes, and so doctors are recommending that patients take a drug which can trigger a condition that drastically lowers quality of life and shortens longevity. Yet the FDA describes the increased risk of developing Type II diabetes while on statins as a risk of "higher blood sugar." That's akin to a Federal Reserve chairman making a speech substituting the word inflation for "an increase in prices."

Statins also can cause liver failure and are linked to auto-immune diseases, among many other potential side effects. Even though the FDA continues to ignore statins' ill effects, ambulance chasing lawyers are paying close attention. Search the internet for "statin lawsuits" and you'll find individual and class-action lawsuits with tragic details on how statins literally ruined people's lives. People in baseline poor health became sicker after developing Type II diabetes. People with rhabdomyolysis developed chronic muscle pain that can only be relieved by oxycodone and are now addicted to opioids.

Yet despite all that, statins are blockbuster drugs with protected status by the FDA. There are dozens of FDA-approved statins, and newer, more expensive brand name statins are continually approved. Using tricks described earlier, big pharma combines statins with generic Type II diabetes drugs to make expensive brand name drugs for the unfortunate patients who developed Type II diabetes because of statins.

The story of statins is a self-perpetuating cycle: patients look first to doctors to solve their problems rather than looking inward, and doctors use statin "calculators" based on medical guidelines that essentially put any patient over the age of 65 years on a statin, regardless of cholesterol levels. Those statins cause new problems, and patients take those new problems back to their doctors. The FDA turns a blind eye and continually approves new statins. Rinse and repeat.

It would be one brand of evil if all the FDA's actions were explained by the promise of future personal gain. After all, bureaucrats at the FDA are rewarded handsomely for their loyalty by big pharma, and personal greed is a common explanation for malfeasance. Case in point: less than a year after facilitating the emergency use authorization for Moderna's COVID-19 vaccine, FDA commissioner Stephen Hahn became the Chief Medical Officer at Flagship Pioneering, the venture capital firm that helped launch Moderna.

But many other FDA blunders have no apparent financial motive and presumably result from sheer incompetence.

The drug class called angiotensin-converting-enzyme (ACE) inhibitors is a perfect example of the FDA's carelessness and inattention to products which do not have a big pharma payoff. ACE inhibitors are prescribed to treat high blood pressure and are cheap, generic drugs. No drug company makes a profit off ACE inhibitors anymore (unless ACE inhibitors are combined with another drug into an expensive combination pill). Theoretically, FDA regulators should feel free to truly weigh the risks and benefits of ACE inhibitors, including their potential life-threatening side effects.

Unfortunately, that is not the case. While the FDA has slapped a "black box" warning on ACE inhibitors advising against their use in pregnant women due to the risk of birth defects, that warning misses ACE inhibitors' gravest side effect, a life-threatening type of allergic reaction.

All drugs carry the risk of an allergic reaction because they are foreign material being introduced into the body. Fortunately, most drug reactions are confined to hives or an upset stomach. But the potential allergic reaction to ACE inhibitors is much more severe. ACE inhibitors can cause angioedema, which is swelling of the lips, tongue, throat, and eventually the vocal cords. If a person's vocal cords swell big enough, airflow to the lungs will be blocked, leading to asphyxiation. Angioedema is a life-threatening emergency which requires quick treatment, potentially involving inserting a breathing tube to stent open a patient's airway.

The additional problem with angioedema from ACE inhibitors is that it is completely unpredictable. Typical drug reactions occur after the first or second dose, but with ACE inhibitors a patient might take the drug for years before suddenly developing angioedema. Oftentimes the only preceding symptom is a slight tingling feeling in the lips, which could be easily ignored by someone who has been taking ACE inhibitors for a long time.

The FDA would argue that the estimated incidence of angioedema from ACE inhibitors is only 0.1 - 0.7%. Those percentages may seem trivial until you consider that millions of Americans take ACE inhibitors and that every single case of angioedema can be life-threatening. In my clinical experience, it is not uncommon to see a patient stumble into the ER with swollen lips that literally hang down past their chin. After inserting a breathing tube into one such patient, a colleague turned to me and asked, *"Remind me why the FDA approved this drug?"*

Beyond drug approval, the FDA's incompetence extends to post-marketing surveillance of drug quality and purity. As detailed in the book *Bottle of Lies*, the FDA fails time and time again to prevent such thing as carcinogens from appearing in antacids, shards of glass in insulin vials, and baby formula filled with asbestos. The FDA blames those mishaps on the outsourcing of generic drug manufacturing to overseas factories in China and India where they have no legal or regulatory authority. Yet the FDA cannot even patrol stateside drug manufacturing, including contaminated drugs from EpiPen manufacturer Mylan Pharmaceuticals and tainted doses of Johnson & Johnson COVID-19 vaccines made in Baltimore. And if you're on a medication for low thyroid, but still gaining weight and losing energy, don't trust that the pills you're taking contain any actual thyroid medication. If one looks closely at medical news over the last decade, there is a laundry list of drug recalls (particularly generic drug recalls) due to lack of the active ingredient.

How does the FDA dismiss contamination at drug manufacturing plants and ignore drugs that aren't drugs? Using the process-based mindset of a bureaucracy, the FDA will say with a straight face that they take those matters very seriously. Allegations of improperly handled biohazardous waste and plant workers soiling themselves while handling drugs are taken so seriously that the FDA will write very strongly worded letters to drug companies.

Those letters come in two flavors: "Official Action Indicated" or "Voluntary Action Indicated." Whether a company ends up receiving one versus the other seems to correlate with lobbying activity and/or media attention to the scandal at hand. Voluntary Action Indicated is the equivalent of a traffic cop warning. You are told to slow down, but then you can drive away, never to see that traffic cop again. Voluntary Action Indicated letters are merely suggestions to companies without any scheduled follow-up.

Official Action Indicated letters are the equivalent of a kindergarten teacher's three-strikes warning system. Official Action Indicated means the company will have several chances to right their wrongs with follow-up FDA inspections. A company can fail those repeated inspections and receive more warning letters before ultimately the FDA will restrict a drug's manufacturing. Companies also can lobby to have senior FDA bureaucrats downgrade Official Action Indicated letters to Voluntary Action Indicated letters.

This ridiculous system of enforcement via letters and overall incompetence extends to medical devices, which are also regulated by the FDA. As with drugs, once medical devices get FDA approval to be inserted into people's bodies, the FDA is supposed to review reports of device malfunctions and adverse events. All those adverse events were previously made publicly available through a database called MAUDE (MAUDE is akin to the CDC's VAERS vaccine adverse events database). However, that was likely too much transparency for the FDA's taste, because the FDA switched to a shadow medical device reporting system called Alternative Summary Reporting. From 2016 - 2019, 1.1 million malfunctions and injuries related to medical devices were reported to that secret, internal FDA database, and only deaths deemed *directly* related to device malfunctions were reported to the public MAUDE database. Once again, FDA actions closely track with lobbying or media attention, and an exposé of Alternative Summary Reporting helped put an end to that shadow reporting system in 2019.

While the FDA is lethargic in bringing its regulatory hammer down on drug and medical device manufacturers, the FDA is quite spry when it comes to quashing their competitors. Little wonder that during the COVID-19 pandemic the FDA turned especially pugnacious and litigious.

Early in 2020, when hand sanitizer was in short supply around the world, resourceful liquor distilleries realized they could help relieve the shortages and make money by repurposing their operations to manufacture hand sanitizer. Alcohol distillers don't offer promising future jobs for FDA bureaucrats, and so tucked into 2020's Coronavirus Aid, Relief, and Economic Security (CARES) act was a provision that prevented private companies from switching their usual production lines over to items such as hand sanitizer, masks, and other types of PPE. The fines for violating that provision were a $14,060 Monograph Drug Facility Fee and a $9,373 Contract Manufacturing Organization Facility Fee. Although HHS, reacting to public outrage, ultimately swooped in and directed the FDA to cease enforcement of those fines, a clear message was delivered and the provision had its intended effect – if you're not part of the government-sanctioned corporate oligarchy, don't bother trying to get into the business of profiting off a pandemic.

The COVID-19 pandemic also revealed big pharma's fear of herbal and naturopathic competition, and the lengths to which the FDA will move regulatory heaven and earth to protect expensive prescription drugs. Receiving regulatory scrutiny just like hydroxychloroquine and ivermectin is a little-known immune boosting supplement called N-acetyl cysteine (NAC).

NAC is an antioxidant precursor, meaning it can increase antioxidant levels in the body and has long been used as a supplement for general health and immune support. Consequently, it falls under the FDA's purview but remained out of the spotlight – until COVID-19. Given NAC's immune and antioxidant boosting properties, and the fact that inhaled NAC can break up mucous plugs in the lungs, researchers began to discuss NAC as a potential adjunct for the treatment of COVID-19.

However, NAC will not reap record-setting quarterly profits for big pharma. Therefore, in mid-2020, the FDA fired off a warning letter to several NAC retailers, which has potentially broad-reaching consequences. The FDA's letter stated that because NAC is FDA-approved for use as a drug to treat acetaminophen overdoses, that it cannot also be considered a dietary supplement. The FDA warned that NAC's regulation and distribution therefore falls under the category of an FDA-approved drug, essentially ending free, over-the-counter access to NAC as a supplement or homeopathic remedy.

Even worse, the FDA's reasoning in the warning letter would not just apply to NAC, but also to a host of supplements that double as FDA-approved drugs for the treatment of a variety of ailments (e.g., magnesium, iron, vitamin B12, folate, thiamine, etc.). While there was no immediate regulatory action accompanying the letter, the intended message was clear – stop trying to sell cheap, homeopathic remedies for COVID-19. The government will not approve of or endorse natural methods to combat disease.

Stick with big pharma instead.

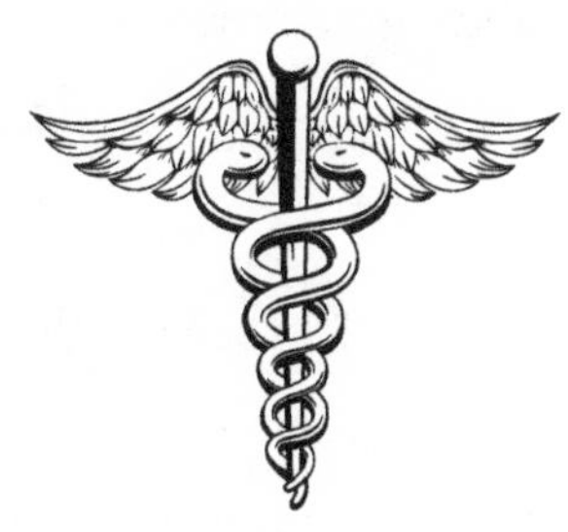

VACCINES: IT DEPENDS ON WHAT THE MEANING OF 'IS' IS

"My message to unvaccinated Americans is this: What more is there to wait for? What more do you need to see? We've made vaccinations free, safe, and convenient.... We've been patient, but our patience is wearing thin."

—President Joseph Biden, September 9, 2021

The systemic ills of the US healthcare system long predate current events. However, COVID-19 has brought them into sharper focus than ever before. The ridiculous and counterproductive way our healthcare system has combatted COVID-19 was merely an extension of how the system previously attacked conditions like high cholesterol and heart disease. If we took the same bright spotlight from COVID-19 and shone it on medical guidelines from the past few decades, many of those recommendations would also whither under scrutiny.

Yet when COVID-19 began this was not readily apparent for most Americans. For most of the public, the gross mismanagement, corruption, and inefficiencies of the medical establishment were out of sight and out of mind, save those with unexpected catastrophic medical events or chronic conditions requiring frequent interface with the healthcare system. But like the Great Recession did for the economy and financial industry, the COVID-19 pandemic brought medicine's decay front and center into Americans' lives. The control that corporate and political powers have over healthcare and individual doctors was broadcast loud and clear into people's homes with press conferences showing US presidents from both political parties side-by-side with big pharma CEOs and directors of the CDC and the NIH. To anyone who could look beyond the right-left political spectrum, the real situation was top versus bottom, with medical decrees coming from corporate oligarchical power backed by an entrenched government bureaucracy.

No issue better represents that system at work than the relentless promotion of COVID-19 vaccines. Encapsulated in the COVID-19 vaccine debacle is the sacrifice of individual liberty in the name of public health, the power of big pharma over its supposed regulatory authorities, the lack of critical thinking of doctors brainwashed by politicized medical societies, and the coercive actions of hospitals and insurance companies, all acting in concert to push a product that does not meet the original definition of a vaccine.

Indeed, governments and regulatory authorities have bent themselves into pretzels, twisting the definition of vaccines to first sell, and then mandate, new and experimental pharmaceutical products that are collectively the biggest blockbuster drugs ever. Worldwide, all the propaganda for and the pushback against COVID-19 vaccines refers collectively to those vaccines as one entity: "the shot," "the jab", or simply "the vaccine." Yet not all COVID-19 vaccines are equal, and some are not even vaccines.

Although the CDC has changed their definition of what a vaccine is, and various governments, the CDC, and the World Health Organization have or will likely change their definition of what fully vaccinated means, the original purpose of vaccines is clear and static. Vaccination prevents disease from happening at all by conferring immunity from infection. Edward Jenner, when developing the smallpox vaccine, was not trying to make infection with smallpox less deadly or have fewer people with smallpox end up in the hospital. Jenner was an innovator aiming to prevent smallpox infection from ever taking hold in people's bodies. Today we don't get smallpox infections that are mild or asymptomatic. We don't get smallpox infections, period. Smallpox has been eradicated from society because of vaccines – that is, except for a few vials stored at the trusty CDC and in Russia (and perhaps elsewhere).

In this sense, COVID-19 vaccines aren't true vaccines. To understand why, it's important to distinguish between exposure and infection. Exposure means your body has some type of contact with a pathogen (e.g., a virus like COVID-19, or a bacterium like pertussis). I personally have been exposed to pertussis on several occasions – unwittingly walking into the room of a coughing, contagious patient who turned out later to have pertussis. Those encounters didn't involve any face masks, meaning the pertussis bacteria flying out with every cough undoubtedly landed inside my mouth and nose. Yet test after test for pertussis always returned negative because as a child I was immunized against pertussis. Decades after my original pertussis immunization, I still have functioning anti-pertussis antibodies. Thus, I have been exposed to pertussis but never infected.

That's because the pertussis vaccine is a real vaccine. Rather than me getting a mild case of whooping cough, the pertussis vaccine saved me from getting whooping cough at all. Officials today reluctantly admit that the COVID-19 vaccines do not prevent you from getting COVID-19, but they stress that those vaccines do make COVID-19 infection less deadly (that assertion is debatable). But the examples of pertussis and of the other traditional childhood vaccinations make it obvious that the COVID-19 vaccines, even if they truly do make infection milder, are akin to prophylactic or therapeutic drugs, not vaccines.

The original childhood vaccines were extraordinarily effective against polio, measles, diphtheria, tetanus, pertussis, and other terrible pathogens. Those traditionally-made childhood vaccines saved countless lives and made pharmaceutical companies a nice sum of money. However, those vaccines were too effective. Although some vaccine immunity wanes in old age, for the most part childhood vaccines confer long-lasting immunity. Therefore, traditional childhood vaccines do not generate repeat customers after the initial series of shots. A few newer vaccines have been produced (e.g., rotavirus, Hepatitis B), but again, same problem. No repeat customers when you make vaccines that confer actual immunity.

In today's corporate world, it is not enough to do something beneficial for society and make a nice sum of money at the same time. You must make obscene gobs of money, more money than last quarter, money that makes your shareholders ultra-rich and happy that their stock portfolio is outpacing inflation, and money that buys power and influence in politics and government. And so along came the flu shot, and the perversion of what it means to be vaccinated.

Influenza, commonly referred to as the flu, has been around since at least Hippocrates' time. Like COVID-19, the flu is a pesky seasonal virus that mutates constantly and can be deadly for the elderly, pregnant women, immunocompromised individuals, or those with serious medical problems. Like COVID-19, there are occasional tragic cases where the flu kills an otherwise healthy individual or a young child.

Pharmaceutical companies realized that the flu infects many people every year and that the flu virus mutates every year. Thus, a new flu vaccine would have to be made and administered every year. That would be a blockbuster drug and a gift that keeps on giving. And so in the 1930s, backed by big pharma money, researchers (including Jonas Salk, future inventor of the first polio vaccine) began trying to make a flu vaccine.

However, attempts at an effective flu vaccine failed for decades. Yet big pharma's push for a flu vaccine continued, even after the 1976 disaster when President Gerald Ford's government rushed a hastily made vaccine against the "Hong Kong flu" into Americans' arms. That vaccine caused hundreds of people to become paralyzed, resulting in an abrupt halt to the nationwide vaccine campaign. Unfortunately, society's collective memory of that debacle did not survive to the COVID-19 pandemic.

Despite the monetary incentive and nearly a century of biomedical advances, we still do not have flu vaccines that provide true immunity against the flu. What today's flu vaccines do is provide transient and modest protection against contracting flu (like a prophylactic drug), and the hopes that if you still get the flu, maybe you'll get less sick (like a therapeutic drug). Why is that so? The flu virus mutates too much and too fast to design a vaccine that is nearly 100% effective. Does that sound familiar?

Perhaps, even in today's modern world, there are some things out of reach of our technology, parts of mother nature, like fast-mutating seasonal viruses, that we cannot conquer. In some cases, we are best advised to develop early therapeutics – like Oseltamivir for the flu, which is somewhat effective, and monoclonal antibodies for COVID-19, which are very effective – and encourage primary prophylaxis via strengthening the immune system and improving health in general.

Yet we see the same script playing out with COVID-19 that played out with the flu. If you think the COVID-19 vaccine madness will stop, consider that flu vaccine development has been trying and failing to contain the flu since the 1930s. But the public health establishment and the media continue to push yearly flu vaccines, and most healthcare and many educational entities mandate the flu shot. Thanks to the backing of the political and medical establishment, the flu vaccine is a $6 billion annual business.

The history of flu vaccines and COVID-19 vaccines diverges at a crucial point. Setting aside that neither function as a real vaccine, there is the key fact that while flu vaccines are still made with traditional vaccine technology (for now), as of this writing all the COVID-19 vaccines available in the US are of the new types of vaccines.

Briefly, traditional vaccines fall into two categories – protein-based and inactivated virus. In protein-based vaccines like the combined diphtheria, tetanus, and pertussis vaccine, a virus protein or pieces of a virus protein are injected into your body. Your immune system recognizes that foreign protein and makes antibodies against it. The goal is for those anti-protein antibodies to block infection if you are exposed to that virus in the future. An inactivated virus vaccine like the combined mumps, measles, and rubella vaccine contains an actual virus particle, chemically neutered so it can't infect you. You are injected with inactivated virus particles and your immune system then makes antibodies against all kinds of proteins on the surface of the virus. In general, inactivated virus vaccines confer excellent and broad-spectrum immunity. Flu vaccines have been made with both protein-based and inactivated virus technology.

But the Pfizer, Moderna, Johnson & Johnson, and AstraZeneca COVID-19 vaccines are neither protein-based nor inactivated virus vaccines. The first two are mRNA vaccines and the last two are adenovirus vector vaccines, and all involve new vaccine technology. Both mRNA and adenovirus vector vaccines inject genetic material into your body, which tricks your cells into making the COVID-19 virus spike protein. Your cells make and release trillions of spike proteins that your immune system is supposed to recognize as foreign and make antibodies against.

Sounds riskier than the traditional methods, right? And anyone who isn't deaf, dumb, or blind has also heard that these new experimental shots have unusual and serious side effects, like myocarditis, blood clots, and strange neurologic reactions. And despite carrying water for big pharma for months after breakthrough infections made the news, the CDC, NIH, and FDA all now admit that the mRNA and adenovirus vector COVID-19 vaccines don't prevent anyone from getting COVID-19.

If you believe the only COVID-19 vaccines out there are mRNA or adenovirus vector vaccines, from those four companies, you are mistaken. In the US and most of the Western World this is true. However, in Russia people can choose between four different COVID-19 vaccines. There is Sputnik V and Sputnik Light, both adenovirus vector vaccines, CoviVac, an inactivated virus vaccine, and EpiVacCorona, a protein-based vaccine. The tour of enemies of the US foreign policy establishment also leads us to China's widely distributed vaccines: Sinovac, a protein-based vaccine, and Sinopharm, an inactivated virus vaccine.

Is this a case of a vaccine Cold War? Are we Westerners flexing our superior technology and the commies simply using old school methods in their backwards ways? Doubtful. Was it faster to make mRNA and adenovirus vector vaccines? No, Sinopharm made its debut in summer of 2020, beating the Western vaccines by several months. And as it turns out, there is a company called Novavax desperately trying to get approval in the US for a protein-based vaccine, and a French company Valneva also struggling to obtain European government approval for an inactivated virus vaccine. Yet as of this writing, curiously the US government paused funding for Novavax and the UK government voted against approving Valneva's vaccine. So why didn't Operation Warp Speed generate FDA emergency use authorizations or full approval for any traditional vaccines?

No one had ever heard of Novavax or Valneva prior to the pandemic, and likely they are still largely unknown to the public and to governments. But Pfizer and Johnson & Johnson are household names with enormous lobbying power. (Moderna, somehow, inserted themselves into the mix, but it is increasingly looking like the chosen sacrificial lamb to atone for vaccine injuries.) The truth is that, as big names in many a mutual fund, if Pfizer and Johnson & Johnson succeed, then all the fat cats win. Probably the best hope for Novavax and Valneva at this point is to be bought out by a big name with financial and political power.

Even before experimental drugs were jabbed into people's arms, the Operation Warp Speed vaccine development program perfectly embodied the corporate and government stranglehold on healthcare. Worldwide, 29 companies were furiously working on developing COVID-19 vaccines as early as February 2020. Congress passed the CARES act in March 2020, authorizing $9.5 billion for COVID-19 vaccine development. Soon thereafter, big pharma began receiving custom handouts because, of course, they couldn't be bothered to put any of their financial skin in the game. Moderna and Johnson & Johnson received vaccine development start-up funds of $954 million and $456 million, respectively. However, it was Pfizer that received the biggest government contract in summer of 2020 (total value $5.97 billion), for a vaccine that hadn't yet received FDA approval.

With payouts and profits secured, the vaccine developers did animal testing while they were jabbing humans for the first time in Phase 1 trials. Then the drug companies combined the Phase 2 and Phase 3 trials. The integrity of those rushed, combined trials in terms of faithfully executing the study design and ensuring data quality has since come into question. It is unclear whether big pharma is following any of the participants from those trials for long-term side effects. It is clear, however, that there is no longer a control group from which to compare the incidence of side effects, as the original control group participants were vaccinated as soon as the brief two-month trials were concluded. All in all, Operation Warp Speed condensed the average 10-year vaccine development timeline into about 10 months.

No matter – the FDA, CDC, and NIH vaccine approvals and endorsements keep rolling in for younger age groups, pregnant women, and booster shots for all. It's also clear that vaccine approvals are timed with events like the 2020 presidential election, and more recently vaccine mandates seem timed to distract from rising inflation. Meanwhile, medical professional societies and individual doctors continue to cover up real and alarming COVID-19 vaccine side effects like myocarditis in young people by labeling those cases as "rare" and "mild."

Individual doctors, hospitals, medical organizations, and governmental agencies have embraced their role in spreading COVID-19 vaccine propaganda. Effective propaganda divides the entire population into two groups – good and evil. According to propaganda, both those groups are completely homogeneous entities, which eliminates any nuance to the debate that might 1) erode the message, and 2) create alliances between people that are supposed to hate each other.

Therefore, those who are unvaccinated against COVID-19 are portrayed as a singular, faceless, and mindless entity. In reality, the unvaccinated are a mix of far right and far left thinkers, naturalists, skeptics, minorities, highly educated clinicians and scientists, people with natural immunity to COVID-19, and others who are critically assessing their individual risks and benefits and deciding not to get a vaccine. Also sympathetic to this group are people who got vaccinated and now regret their choice, or people who were forced into getting a vaccine due to economic circumstances.

Lost in lumping the heterogeneous group of unvaccinated people into one category of obstinate science deniers is how many are "vaccine hesitant" because the COVID-19 vaccines aren't real vaccines? How many people will not take a mRNA or adenovirus vector vaccine, but would consider a protein-based or inactivated virus COVID-19 vaccine? How many people would rather that folks with a low risk tolerance for COVID-19 infection wear N95 masks and leave the rest of us alone? No one knows because no one will bother to ask.

And now, worldwide, doctors, workers, and citizens in general are faced with mandates that whittle their options down to jab or job, and increasingly, jab or second-class citizen. The lack of vaccine choice (not just what type to get, but whether to get one at all) is but one symptom of Western society's greater decline. America and the West are supposed to embody freedom and choice. But just as we have created supply shortages, reduced the stock market to ride the whims of 10 companies, and gutted small businesses in favor of Amazon, so too have our health options been whittled down to jab or job. A BMI of 20 or a deadlift of 405 pounds cannot grant entry into a restaurant, but Pfizer can.

Beyond being barred from entry into restaurants and grocery stores, obtaining affordable health insurance, seeing your children, and making a living, God forbid if you get COVID-19 and are unvaccinated. While the vaccinated can also contract and spread COVID-19, the unvaccinated should expect an uphill battle with conventional doctors at clinics and hospitals and a lot of "I told you so." The COVID-19 virus stopped being the common enemy shortly after the pandemic started. The real battle lines were drawn between individuals who think for themselves and the compliant.

But even if you comply and get the COVID-19 vaccine, there is no legal recourse for you if you suffer adverse effects. A longstanding federal statute protects pharmaceutical companies from liability for vaccine-related injuries or deaths. Individual physicians were granted immunity from liability related to administering COVID-19 vaccines by a March 2020 declaration from the Secretary of Health and Human Services, coinciding with the launch of Operation Warp Speed. And even if one could sue, no amount of money can heal injuries or bring back the dead. Therefore, more important than the legal system making someone fiscally whole after an injury is not being damaged by biomedical tyranny in the first place.

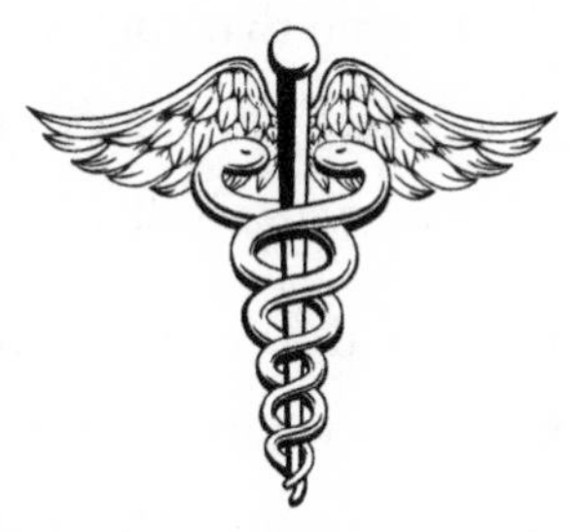

CONCLUSION: WHAT CAN WE DO?

"The deviation of man from the state in which he was originally placed by nature seems to have proved to him a prolific source of diseases."

—Edward Jenner

At this point, some readers may want to run away from our US healthcare system. I completely understand. There is no easy fix. The bureaucrats and corporations described here will not disappear just because there's a new Congress or a new President. And given the mindset of doctors graduating from medical schools and the politicization of the entire healthcare system during the COVID-19 pandemic, the likelihood is that medicine will move farther away from health and more towards a preoccupation with "social justice."

Therefore, I would argue that the pressing question for today is not how do we elect new blood into the establishment system, but what can we as individuals do instead?

One of the few good things to come out of the COVID-19 pandemic is far greater clarity on where institutions stand. Millions of people understand now that hospitals and medical organizations don't work for patients, but rather are slaves to corporate and governmental handlers. Perhaps some also realize that it is immaterial whether in the future the US healthcare system moves toward a full corporate welfare state or to a single payer system, since both are government-subsidized, thereby guaranteeing an inefficient and corrupt system that does not improve health.

It would seem that to bring down the current regime and rebuild a functional healthcare system would take an act of God, an occurrence that may not happen in our lifetimes.

Fortunately, it is now easier to identify which states virtue signal while sending COVID-positive patients into nursing homes to seed deadly outbreaks, and which states block federal government overreach into what should be personalized patient care.

In fact, one of the best options is simply to live in an area where healthcare organizations and individual doctors are permitted to freely practice medicine rather than robotically follow mandates and edicts. As hard as relocating may be, in a free environment there is a better chance of finding a doctor who will evaluate each patient as a unique individual and treat him like a fellow human being.

For notwithstanding much that appears in this book, there remains a critical mass of good and even great doctors whose primary purpose is to help others. Post-COVID-19 vaccine mandates, it's become easier than ever to identify the doctors and other clinicians who are independent and critical thinkers – many have been pushed out of big hospitals and affiliated clinics and are looking to strike out on their own.

This makes the current medical environment ripe for the development of parallel and decentralized healthcare system. To avoid federal and local mandates, many doctors (and nurses, nurse practitioners, physician assistants, emergency medical technicians, and other medical professionals) could deploy their hard-earned skillsets as small, independently owned businesses serving the many Americans fed up with being treated as nameless, faceless patients by the establishment healthcare system.

Even without radical state or federal legislation, most current regulations allow for house calls for working parents and busy families, concierge care, telemedicine, and even the return of the town or neighborhood general practitioner. If medical providers undercut insurance premiums and co-pays by setting realistic fee-for-service prices, patients could pay outright for affordable and high-quality care offered in an alternative system without having to haggle with insurance companies. At the same time, online scheduling systems make connecting with patients easier than ever and lessen the need for medical administrative staff.

What would further facilitate this model of decentralized medical care is a readjustment of income needs and expectations by doctors. But that may only be possible in the long-term if the bubble finally bursts on the inflated price tag of medical school and with decreases in medical student debt.

The ideal solution for medical education is to return to a true apprenticeship system, towards something similar to how electricians and other tradesmen are trained. I would propose one intensive year in the classroom followed by several years as a hybrid apprentice/resident doctor working one-on-one with an experienced doctor in the desired field of practice, with rotations with other doctors of different specialties sprinkled in for breadth of knowledge. The MBBS degree in Europe condenses undergraduate and graduate medical studies. There is no reason we can't do the same in the US, reducing the student debt burden that drives the dysfunctional incentives that exist for medical students here.

Following such an apprenticeship, doctors would feel emboldened and encouraged to "hang a shingle" and start their own practice. Independent practice is still possible today for primary care doctors and in some specialties such as rheumatology, neurology, and pediatrics. Other, more procedural-based specialties, such as cardiology, anesthesiology, and gastroenterology will still require some affiliation with a hospital or surgery center.

As for emergency medicine, over 70% of the patients treated in ERs do not have an actual emergency. If primary care doctors were better-trained, more available, and offered a reasonable pricing scheme, a small number of hospital-based emergency physicians would be able to focus on the true emergencies like car accidents, strokes, and heart attacks.

Legislative action at the state level would greatly facilitate and expedite this alternative model of healthcare. State medical boards should cross-reference their medical licensing requirements and figure out a way to authorize the practice of medicine from providers in adjacent states. States should also allow for faster, cheaper, and easier creation of professional limited liability companies, not just for doctors but also for nurses, nurse practitioners, physician assistants, and other types of clinicians. State legislatures should also expand the scope of practice for those clinicians so they can similarly strike out on their own and increase the supply of readily available medical care. (Recall that the AMA is dumping cash to stop precisely this – it's long past time to put an end to the AMA protecting a cabal of entitled doctors.)

With more options for primary care, prices for medical services would fall and patients could get by with catastrophic healthcare insurance coverage only, minimizing how much hard-earned money is fed into a corrupt system.

I often say that the best medical advice I can give is to not need medical advice. By this I mean that the greatest change we can make in healthcare, beyond improving the supply side, is to radically decrease the *demand* for healthcare. Simply put, America must get healthy.

Alongside the medical establishment is the synergistic oligopoly of big agriculture that has made the average American obese and unhealthy. Just as we should reject the advice of fat cardiologists, we should reject the dogma that has people voraciously consuming vegetable oils and fake meat. We should also demand a higher performance level from our bodies by being active and strong. For each of us this is our personal responsibility – it is our individual lives at stake.

The goal should be to need as little healthcare as possible – that is the best way to defeat the current system. Rather than spend disposable income on co-pays for useless annual physicals and harmful statin prescriptions, people must understand how essential it is to spend their money on high-quality, nutrient-rich foods, gym memberships, and other ways to access exercise.

As with new small business models of healthcare delivery, local healthcare insurance cooperatives could encourage healthy behavior and be greatly facilitated by state legislation. Such cooperatives could require certain health standards that demand individual responsibility. Nor would this insurance model necessarily penalize people with pre-existing conditions. I'd much rather share in a health insurance cooperative with an asthmatic who takes care to follow an anti-inflammatory diet or a bodybuilding Type I diabetic than someone with "no medical conditions" save a BMI of 30 because they can't resist fast food.

Of course, that's not to say that healthcare won't be needed. Whether from aging, chronic conditions, or emergent care needed during a pandemic, at some point in our lives we will all require healthcare. The type and amount needed, however, depends on our baseline health.

The urgent need to optimize individual health and nutrition has never been more tragically illustrated than during the COVID-19 pandemic, when it became clear how dramatically obesity increased the risk of dying from the virus.

When it comes to delivering more involved care, small, independent hospitals could build off a decentralized primary care system and operate in the manner that independent surgery centers operate today. Known officially as ambulatory surgery centers (ASCs), those centers employ surgeons, anesthesiologists, nurses, and medical technicians and offer a wide variety of procedures and surgeries without the hassle of going to a hospital. In fact, many ASCs are independent of big corporate and academic hospital chains.

However, there still will be a need for big hospitals that specialize in the most complex conditions. Fields like oncology and transplant medicine have dramatically evolved over the past few decades to provide life-saving care for otherwise fatal conditions. Removing access to highly specialized care would destroy one of the few benefits of our hyper-specialized healthcare system.

Still, in the long run, a healthier population will shrink demand for such niche services. That shrinking demand will leave true charity cases like infants who need surgery for congenital heart defects and adults suffering from rare and deadly diseases. Those large medical expenses should be thought of as investments in our community and covered in full by a benevolent government that truly cares about its citizens.

The path forward for healthcare I propose necessarily raises the issue of a high trust society. All parties involved in any medical encounter must be assured that the end goal is not a prescription or a bill, but rather an honest assessment of the situation rooted in mutual goodwill. Rather than chasing empty consumption, we should chase real human connection.

Before accusing me of being naïve, it's important to know that within memory, that was very much the basis on which American healthcare operated. Until the 1960s, medical malpractice litigation was extremely uncommon in the US. In fact, while today the cost of medical malpractice insurance is one of the major barriers to doctors opening independent practices, prior to 1960, most doctors had never heard of such insurance. Nor is it a coincidence that the corporatization and consolidation of healthcare took off at the same time medical malpractice lawsuits did.

I don't claim to have the answers for all of healthcare's problems. The CDC's contradictory policies, the NIH's funding of selective research, and the FDA's dysfunctional drug approval process are just a few examples of massive issues that are intertwined with the more systemic ills in America. Our healthcare and greater sociopolitical system were already in the late stages of decline prior to COVID-19, and the pandemic only laid bare and accelerated the extent of that deterioration.

But there is no question that the place to start is with a return to the independent practitioner model built on a healthier, localized, high trust society, and the short-term solutions I have proposed can be achieved right now. Literally thousands of doctors, nurse practitioners, and physician assistants were outraged by the medical establishment's mistreatment of COVID-19 patients, and many set up telemedicine operations to deliver care that included *verboten* prescriptions such as ivermectin. Regular citizens became aware that they could directly order drugs like ivermectin from overseas pharmacies, circumventing the FDA's politicized drug approvals.

In short, countless patients and their families are ready to leave a system which allots fifteen minutes for a primary care appointment to discuss six topics, and ready to reject doctors who wait an average of eleven seconds before interrupting a patient.

Most importantly, people are beginning to realize the current healthcare system, rather than provide care, regularly delivers harm. Before the COVID-19 pandemic, medical errors were the third-leading cause of death in the US. Now we are only scratching the surface of the harm done by the pandemic, with reports piling into the CDC's VAERS database of adverse events and deaths "associated" with COVID-19 vaccines, and a recently released document with 1,291 potential side effects.

As tech entrepreneurs would pitch it to venture capitalists, the time is ripe for disruption.

In closing as a physician who has witnessed the crash of a dysfunctional and politicized system into a pandemic, I feel compelled to offer some medical advice. Seeming obvious as it sounds, we must each cultivate and cherish our health the way parents do their children. Engage in your own independent science and read as much as you can while thinking critically. What health philosophies are internally consistent and don't contradict what you see in real life? What works for you in practice?

Feel emboldened with your knowledge to be disagreeable in speaking with the doctors who repeat what you recognize as industry-sponsored talking points. Seek out like-minded friends and medical practitioners who will help you improve yourself rather than reinforce bad habits. Most importantly, do not *ever* give in to something that your instinct says is wrong for your health. Although corporations and government may control the doctors and the healthcare system, you still control your health.

And as Virgil said, "the greatest wealth is health." With strong bodies and independent minds, together we can forge a system which truly cares for health.

SUGGESTED READINGS

NUTRITION

Deep Nutrition: Why Your Genes Need Traditional Food. By Cate Shanahan.

Dumping Iron: How to Ditch This Secret Killer and Reclaim Your Health. By P.D. Mangan.

FITNESS

Becoming a Supple Leopard: The Ultimate Guide to Resolving Pain, Preventing Injury, and Optimizing Athletic Performance. By Kelly Starrett with Glen Cordoza.

The New Rules of Lifting for Women: Lift Like a Man, Look Like a Goddess. By Lou Schuler, Cassandra Forsythe, and Alwyn Cosgrove.

Maximum Strength: Get Your Strongest Body In 16 Weeks with the Ultimate Weight-Training Program. By Eric Cressey and Matt Fitzgerald.

GLOSSARY

AAMC – Association of American Medical Colleges

AAP – American Academy of Pediatrics

ACE inhibitors – Angiotensin-converting-enzyme inhibitors

ACGME – Accreditation Council for Graduate Medical Education

ACPeds – American College of Pediatricians

AHA – American Hospital Association

AHRQ – Agency for Healthcare Research and Quality

AMA – American Medical Association

AMPAC – American Medical Political Action Committee

APRN – Advanced Practice Registered Nurses

ASC – Ambulatory Surgical Center

CDC – Centers for Disease Control and Prevention

CEO – Chief Executive Officer

CFO – Chief Financial Officer

CIA – Central Intelligence Agency

CMO – Chief Medical Officer

CMS – Centers for Medicare and Medicaid Services

CON – Certificates of Need

DDT - dichlorodiphenyltrichloroethane

DO – Doctor of Osteopathy

Doctor – physician, a medical doctor

Doctors Without Borders – aka Médecins Sans Frontières

ECFMG – Education Commission for Foreign Medical Graduates

ED – Emergency Department, also known as Emergency Room (ER)

EHR – Electronic Health Record, also known as the electronic medical record (EMR)

EMT – Emergency Medical Technician

EMTALA – Emergency Medical Treatment & Labor Act

FDA – Food and Drug Administration

FSMB – Federation of State Medical Boards

HCAHPS – Hospital Consumer Assessment of Healthcare Providers and Systems

HHS – Health and Human Services

HRSA – Health Resources and Services Administration

HIV – Human Immunodeficiency Virus

ICU – Intensive Care Unit

LCME – Liaison Committee on Medical Education

Note: LCME® is a registered trademark of the Association of American Medical Colleges and the American Medical Association.

LSD – lysergic acid diethylamide

MBBS – Bachelor of Medicine, Bachelor of Surgery

MCAT – Medical College Admission Test

MD – Medical Doctorate

MK-ULTRA – Cold War-era CIA program

NBME – National Board of Medical Examiners

NIAID – National Institute for Allergy and Infectious Diseases

NIH – National Institutes of Health

NIMH – National Institute of Mental Health

NNU – National Nurses United

NRMP – National Residency Matching Program

NSF – National Science Foundation

OHSA – Occupational Health and Safety Administration

PBM – Pharmacy Benefit Managers

PCORI – Patient-Centered Outcomes Research Institute

PPE – Personal Protective Equipment

Physician – a medical doctor, a doctor

R&D – research and development

STD – sexually transmitted disease

STEMI – ST segment elevation myocardial infarction

UN – United Nations

US – United States

USAMRIID - United States Army Medical Research Institute of Infectious Diseases

USMLE – United States Medical Licensing Examination

US PHS – United States Public Health Service

VA – Veterans Affairs

VAERS – Vaccine Adverse Events Reporting System

VBP – Value Based Purchasing

REFERENCES

INTRODUCTION

Many scientists believe that COVID-19 primarily damages blood vessels.

Nuovo GJ, et al. Endothelial cell damage is the central part of COVID-19 and a mouse model induced by injection of the S1 subunit of the spike protein. *Annals of Diagnostic Pathology*. 2021;51:151682.

Two-thirds of Americans in a 2021 survey said they trusted the US healthcare system.

Surveys of Trust in the US Healthcare System. ABIM Foundation. June 2, 2021.

59% of respondents to a 2021 poll said they gained confidence in doctors during the COVID-19 pandemic. MedCity News. August 17, 2021.

MEDICAL EDUCATION & TRAINING: FAILING FORWARD

Most of the American public admires and has faith in physicians. Pew Research Center, August 2019, "Trust and Mistrust in Americans' Views of Scientific Experts."

Medical School Accreditation Standards

Liaison Committee on Medical Education (LCME®). Functions and Structure of a Medical School. Standards for Accreditation of Medical Education Programs Leading to the MD Degree & Data Collection Instrument. Published October 2021 for surveys in the 2022-23 Academic Year.

Graduating Medical Student Survey

Association of American Medical Colleges 2021 Medical School Graduation Questionnaire.

Copyright October 2021, Association of American Medical Colleges and American Medical Association.

US medical schools accept between 1% - 20% of their applicants.

2022 statistics from Accepted.com

For students applying to medical schools, their acceptance rate is around 40%.

American Association of Medical Colleges (AAMC) report on Applicants, Matriculants, Enrollment, and Graduates of U.S. MD-Granting Medical Schools, 2012-2013 through 2021-2022.

At the time of the US invasion of Grenada in 1983, the St. George's University School of Medicine had about 700 American medical students and generated between 10-15% of Grenada's national GDP.

SOF Mag. Operation Urgent Fury, the 1983 Invasion of Grenada. October 25, 2016.

More 'prestigious' Caribbean medical schools accept between 40-44% of their applicants.

Ingeniusprep.com. A Guide to Caribbean Medical Schools. August 27, 2019.

Caribbean medical school graduates have lower board exam pass rates and a harder time matching into residency than stateside medical school graduates.

US News & World Report. What to Know About Caribbean Medical Education. January 13, 2020.

The AAMC reports an overall medical student graduation rate of 96%.

AAMC Data Snapshot. Graduation Rates and Attrition Rates of U.S. Medical Students. October 2021.

Medical school grades are pass-fail.

AMA. How do Medical Schools Use Pass-Fail Grading? January 9, 2020.

95% of hospital residency positions are filled during The Match.

The Redesign of the Matching Market for American Physicians: Some Engineering Aspects of Economic

Design. Alvin E. Roth and Elliott Peranson. *The American Economic Review*. September 1999.

ACGME resident duty hours restrictions adopted in 2003.

Philibert I, Friedmann P, Williams WT, for the members of the ACGME Work Group on Resident Duty Hours. New Requirements for Resident Duty Hours. JAMA. 2002;288(9):1112–1114.

Resident duty hour restrictions increase the number of patient hand-offs.

Christopher DeRienzo, et al. Handoffs in the Era of Duty Hours Reform. *Academic Medicine*. April 2012. Vol 87, Issue 4, p 403-410.

Patient handoffs are a major risk factor for serious medical errors.

Sentinel event data: root causes by event type. The Joint Commission, March 19, 2014.

ACGME Resident Milestones

The Milestones Guidebook. Version 2020. Copyright Accreditation Council for Graduate Medical Education (ACGME).

ACGME Milestones for Internal Medicine Residents.

Internal Medicine Milestones: The Accreditation Council for Graduate Medical Education. Implementation Date:

July 1, 2021. Copyright Accreditation Council for Graduate Medical Education (ACGME).

Between 71-78% of medical school graduates completed residency within 4 years and the overall number of residency programs in the US is increasing.

AAMC 2019 State Physician Workforce Data Report.

NPDB malpractice payment statistics in text were current as of 2021.

Of malpractice claims paid out between 1986-2010 reported to the NPDB, 28.6% were for diagnostic errors, and 41% of those diagnostic errors resulted in the patient's death.

Saber Tehrani AS, et al. 25-Year summary of US malpractice claims for diagnostic errors 1986-2010: an analysis from the National Practitioner Data Bank. *British Medical Journal Quality & Safety*. 2013;22(8):672-80.

A study of primary care physicians' hypothetical response to a medical error involving a cancer patient revealed that the majority of physicians surveyed would not admit the error to the patient.

Mazor K, et al. Primary care physicians' willingness to disclose oncology errors involving multiple providers to patients. *British Medical Journal Quality & Safety.* 2016;25:787-795.

HOSPITAL ADMINISTRATORS: THE PETER PRINCIPLE

Story of Olga Matievskaya

ProPublica. A Nurse Bought Protective Supplies for Her Colleagues Using GoFundMe. The Hospital Suspended Her. April 7, 2020.

US government studies on expired N-95 efficacy.

National Personal Protective Technology Laboratory Beyond Shelf Life/Stockpiled Assessment Reports. 2020.

A hospital's administrators stayed quiet about staff who fell ill with COVID-19.

The LA Times. "One by one, nurses got coronavirus at a Silicon Valley hospital while management kept quiet." April 10, 2020.

New York State called in national guard to fill healthcare worker shortage during the pandemic.

New York Daily News. Hochul orders National Guard to fill N.Y. hospital shortages caused by staffers not vaccinated against COVID. September 27, 2021.

The Peter Principle

The Peter Principle: Why Things Always go Wrong. Laurence J. Peter and Raymond Hull. Harper Business, 2014.

Between 1975-2010, the number of physicians in the US grew by 150%, and healthcare administrative positions grew by 3,200%.

Becker's Hospital Review. "Growth of healthcare administrators outpaced physicians, increasing 3,200% between 1975-2010. November 9, 2017.

During Hurricane Katrina, many hospitals in the New Orleans region lost power and had their backup generators fail due to flooding.

Gray BH, Hebert K. Hospitals in Hurricane Katrina: challenges facing custodial institutions in a disaster. *Journal of Healthcare for the Poor and Underserved.* 2007;18(2):283-98.

Swine flu after action reports and lack of preventative action post-swine flu.

Relias Media. Emergency Medicine Reports. "The Next Pandemic: Hospital Management." December 13, 2015.

Individual departments at hospitals waste millions of dollars a year on medical supplies.

ProPublica. "What Hospitals Waste." March 9, 2017.

&

Zygourakis CC, et al. Operating room waste: disposable supply utilization in neurosurgical procedures. *Journal of Neurosurgery*. 2017;126(2):620-625.

The drug shortage crisis in the US.

Ventola CL. The drug shortage crisis in the United States: causes, impact, and management strategies. *Pharmacy & Therapeutics.* 2011;36(11):740-757.

Hospital runs out of life-saving medication.

ProPublica. "She Needed Lifesaving Medication, but the Only Hospital in Town Did Not Have It." July 1, 2020.

COVID-19 ventilators were thrown away.

Local 10 News Miami. "Why are new ventilators being trashed in a Miami-Dade landfill?" April 19, 2021.

Doctors are naïve about finance.

The Wall Street Journal. "Telling Doctors What Ails Them." April 14, 2015.

HOSPITALS: FIRST WORLD PARASITES

Private equity firms are buying hospitals.

ProPublica. "These Hospitals Pinned Their Hopes on Private Management Companies. Now They're Deeper in Debt." June 4, 2020.

HCA's 2021 third quarter profits were $2.3 billion.

Becker's Hospital Review. HCA's profit more than triples to $2.3B in Q3. October 22, 2021.

HCA has been investigated for unnecessary cardiac procedures.

The New York Times. Hospital Chain Inquiry Cited Unnecessary Cardiac Work. August 6, 2012.

HCA was engaged in $1.7 billion in Medicare fraud, with implication of direct involvement by Rick Scott.

Tampa Bay Times. HCA Whistleblower revives claim that Scott knew of fraud. October 6, 2014.

Bill Frist is related to the founding members of HCA.

Slate. Frist's Real HCA Scandal. September 27, 2005.

National Nurses United union filed a complaint in 2020 with the federal Occupational Health and Safety Administration (OHSA) alleging that HCA hospitals in 17 states were engaged in unsafe practices related to COVID-19.

National Nurses United Press Release. Nurses seek OSHA sanctions on HCA. August 24, 2020.

Tenet was fined $900 million by Medicare for fraud.

Insider Exclusive. America's "Hospital of Horrors" – Tenet Healthcare – the $400 Million Dollar Health Care Fraud Story. October 25, 2017.

A study from Washington state estimated 600,000 patients in a single year were subject to an unnecessary medical procedure.

Washington Health Alliance. First, Do No Harm. February 2018.

A study from Virginia estimated that $586 million was spent on unnecessary medical care in one year.

Low-Cost, High-Volume Health Services Contribute The Most to Unnecessary Health Spending. *Health Affairs*. Vol 36, No 10. October 2017.

A hospital charged $1,877 to pierce a 5-year-old's ears.

ProPublica. A Hospital Charged $1,877 to Pierce a 5-Year-Old's Ears. This is Why Health Care Costs So Much. November 28, 2017.

The then-President of the Association of American Physicians and Surgeons in 2018 wrote, "One of my patients received an invoice of around $100,000 for a hysterectomy, of which $68,000 was for the use of a robot."

Albert L. Fischer, MD. Corruption in Medicine. *Journal of American Physicians and Surgeons*. Winter 2018 ed. Vol 23, No 4.

The value of the nonprofit hospital tax exemption was $24.6 billion in 2011.

The Value of the Nonprofit Hospital Tax Exemption was $24.6 Billion in 2011. *Health Affairs*. Vol 34, No 7. July 2015.

Charity care hospitals chase after indigent patients with inflated bills devoid of discounts. ProPublica. Nonprofit Hospitals Almost Never Gave Discounts to Poor Patients During Collections, Documents Show. December 4, 2020.

Some charity care applications include questions about the patient's car.

The Washington Post. Free or Discounted Care is Available at Some Hospitals But They Don't Make it Easy. October 11, 2019.

Charity care hospitals have hired their own bill collectors.

ProPublica. The Nonprofit Hospital that Makes Millions, Owns a Collection Agency and Relentlessly Sues the Poor. June 27, 2019.

Non-profit hospitals have used revenue in excess of expenses to fund 7-figure executive pay, bonuses, lavish conferences, private jets to fly to said lavish conferences, and even offshore bank accounts.

Medical Economics. How nonprofit hospitals get away with the biggest rip off in America. January 17, 2020.

Medicaid and Medicare insure about 40% Americans.

From Statista.com, February 2022.

At times, CMS reimburses hospitals pennies on the dollar or outright denies reimbursement.

American Hospital Association Fact Sheet. Underpayment by Medicare and Medicaid. January 2021.

CMS Hospital Rankings

Medicare.gov - Care Compare. Available at: https://www.medicare.gov/care-compare/

Hospitals have gamed CMS' mortality metric by keeping vegetative patients alive just past the due dates of their CMS reports.

ProPublica. "It's Very Unethical": Audio Shows Hospital Kept Vegetative Patient on Life Support to Boost Survival Rates. October 3, 2019.

The Journal of the American Medical Association (AMA) published a study refuting that HCAHPS pain scores were associated with more opioid prescriptions.

Lee HS, et al. Postoperative opioid prescribing and the pain scores on Hospital Consumer Assessment of Healthcare Providers and Systems survey. *Journal of the American Medical Association*. 2017;317(19):2013-2015.

Through the VBP, CMS can turn a $10,000 charge from the hospital to a $200 bill from CMS to the hospital.

CMS Hospital-Acquired Conditions Reduction Program as of February 2022.

Effective January 1, 2022, doctors will receive extra CMS reimbursement if they create and implement an anti-racism plan.

Medicare Program; CY 2022 Payment Policies. Federal Register Vol 86, No 221. Issued November 19, 2021.

US News & World Report Best Hospital Rankings

US News & World Report FAQs: How and Why We Rank and Rate Hospitals. December 7, 2021. Available at: https://health.usnews.com/health-care/best-hospitals/articles/faq-how-and-why-we-rank-and-rate-hospitals

The Joint Commission has four levels of stroke accreditation: comprehensive stroke center, thrombectomy-capable stroke center, primary stroke center, and acute stroke ready hospital.

The Joint Commission© Advanced Stroke Certifications.

The Joint Commission advertises on its website that, "We certify 10 times the number of Acute Stroke Ready Hospitals as the competition."

The Joint Commission.© Acute Stroke Ready Hospital Certification. Accessed February 2022. Available at: https://www.jointcommission.org/accreditation-and-certification/certification/certifications-by-setting/hospital-certifications/stroke-certification/advanced-stroke/certification-for-acute-stroke-ready-hospital/

MEDICAL PROFESSIONAL ORGANIZATIONS: THE SKY IS LAVENDAR!

There is an increased risk of a transfusion reaction if a male receives blood from a female.

Caram-Deelder, Camila et al. "Association of Blood Transfusion From Female Donors With and Without a History of Pregnancy With Mortality Among Male and Female Transfusion Recipients." *Journal of the American Medical Association.* 2017;318(15):1471-1478.

A JAMA review in April 2020 treated both hydroxychloroquine and Remdesivir fairly in describing their relative risks and benefits, including side effects, costs, and availability

Sanders JM, et al. Pharmacologic Treatments for Coronavirus Disease 2019 (COVID-19): A Review. *Journal of the American Medical Association.* 2020;323(18):1824–1836.

JAMA editorial on the hydroxychloroquine and its 'misuse.'

Saag MS. Misguided Use of Hydroxychloroquine for COVID-19: The Infusion of Politics Into Science. *Journal of the American Medical Association.* 2020;324(21):2161–2162.

Some medical providers, including the WHO, have warned about adverse effects from Remdesivir.

NBC News. Remdesivir shouldn't be used on hospitalized Covid-19 patients, WHO advises. November 19, 2020.

JAMA research paper concluding that a healthy diet should not contain more than 4 eggs per week.

Brown HB, et al. Design of Practical Fat-Controlled Diets: Foods, Fat Composition, and Serum Cholesterol Content. *Journal of the American Medical Association.* 1966;196(3):205–213.

JAMA editorial describing egg yolks vibrant color as "betraying the offending cholesterol."

The Martyred Meal. *Journal of the American Medical Association.* 1966;198(13):1362–1363.

The AMA advocated for mandatory smallpox vaccinations.

The Progressive Era's Health Reform Movement: A Historical Dictionary. By Ruth Clifford Engs. Praeger, 2003.

The AMA supports mandatory COVID-19 vaccinations.

AMA President Gerald E. Harmon, M.D., statement on Supreme Court opinions on COVID-19 vaccination and testing, January 13, 2022.

The AMA supports gun control legislation.

AMA Press Release. AMA recommends new, commonsense policies to prevent gun violence. June 12, 2018.

The AMA supported banning tobacco products.

The New York Times. AMA Votes to seek total ban on advertising tobacco products. December 11, 1985.

AMPAC's political donations are biased leftward.

AMPAC. The 2020 Cycle AMPAC Election Report.

AMPAC lobbied for the Affordable Care Act.

AMA. 7 major downsides if the ACA is overturned by the Supreme Court. October 30, 2020.

Most physicians are either opposed to or lukewarm towards the Affordable Care Act.

MedicusFirm. Annual Practice Preference and Relocation Survey: 2020.

The AMA Advocacy in Action 2020 report.

AMA. AMA advocacy 2020-2021 efforts. November 2021.

AMA's 2021 resource document, "Advancing Health Equity: A Guide to Language, Narrative, and Concepts"

AMA and AAMC. Advancing Health Equity: A Guide to Language, Narrative and Concepts. 2021.

Medical schools are adopting curriculums that mirror the recommendations of the "Advancing Health Equity: A Guide to Language, Narrative, and Concepts" resource guide.

City Journal. A blueprint for woke medicine. December 22, 2021.

As of 2016, the AMA's membership was 235,000, comprising only about 17% of all US doctors. In the 1950s, 75% of US doctors were AMA members.

Mother Jones. The AMA Represents Only About One-sixth of All Doctors. December 27, 2016.

AMA opposes scope of practice expansion legislation.

AMA. AMA successfully fights scope of practice expansions that threaten patient safety. November 11, 2021.

APRNs help alleviate workforce shortages in primary care (especially in rural areas) and can lower healthcare costs.

Fierce Healthcare. 'Turf wars' heat up: Nurses fire back at American Medical Association's stand on independent practice. November 20, 2017.

AAP statement: "As we noted in a landmark statement on the Impact of Racism on Child and Adolescent Health in August of 2019…"

AAP Blueprint for Children. 2020.

The AAP has Advocacy Training Modules.

AAP Advocacy Training Modules. Accessed February 2022. Available at: https://services.aap.org/en/advocacy/advocacy-training-modules/

AAP – Human Rights Campaign Resource Document on Transgender Care.

Human Rights Campaign. Supporting & Caring for Transgender Children. September 2016.

Glenn Beck response to ACPeds statement on transgender care.

GlennBeck.com. American College of Pediatricians: Pushing Gender Ideology Is 'Child Abuse.' May 16, 2016.

Media reports about the AAP – ACPeds disagreement characterized the AAP as prestigious.

Snopes.com. Did American pediatricians issue a statement that transgenderism is 'child abuse'? May 20, 2016.

Hillary Rodham Clinton speech at AAP Convention in 2014.

AAP YouTube channel. Hillary Rodham Clinton Unveils Early Literacy Toolkit at American Academy of Pediatrics Conference. Accessed February 2022. Available at: https://www.youtube.com/watch?v=AsvJ0ELsegE

Vice News segment on a Los Angeles ER doctor.

Vice News YouTube channel. Fighting on the Front-line's of LA's COVID Catastrophe. Accessed February 2022. Available at: https://www.youtube.com/watch?v=pUN0YlIvjk8

Physicians from Doctors Without Borders have been abducted from the Congo.

Doctors Without Borders. DRC: Abducted MSF Team Member Found Unharmed. September 1, 2014.

Physicians from Doctors Without Borders have been shot while in Afghanistan

Huffington Post. Doctors Without Borders staff shot while fleeing Kunduz hospital, report finds. November 6, 2015.

The FSMB cites wellness and burnout as important issues for physicians.

Federation of State Medical Boards. Physician Wellness and Burnout. April 2018.

In 2021, the Federation of State Medical Boards (FSMB) and the National Board of Medical Examiners (NBME) announced that the Step 1 United States Medical Licensing Examination (USMLE) would become pass / fail.

USMLE. USMLE Step 1 Transition to Pass/Fail Only Score Reporting. September 2021.

CDC's Top 10 list of public health accomplishments.

CDC MMWR Weekly. Ten Great Public Health Achievements – United States, 1900-1999. 1999;48(12); 241-243.

Sunscreens that were supposed to prevent skin cancer contained carcinogens.

CBS News. Carcinogen found in some popular sunscreens and after-sun products including Neutrogena, tests show. June 5, 2021.

The fluorine added to our drinking water and toothpaste to prevent tooth decay is linked to thyroid problems.

Peckham S, Awofeso N. Water fluoridation: a critical review of the physiological effects of ingested fluoride as a public health intervention. *Scientific World Journal.* February 26, 2014.

Chantix has been linked to cancer.

Drug Watch. Chantix Recalled over Potential Cancer Risk. September 23, 2021.

Harvard T.H. Chan School of Public Health MPH curriculum.

Harvard T.H. Chan School of Public Health. MPH Generalist Curriculum for Fall 2021 start. Accessed February 2022.

The biostatistical methods of today's clinical trials are extremely complex.

Bowalekar S. Adaptive designs in clinical trials. *Perspectives in Clinical Research.* 2011;2(1):23-7.

The CDC's concern with smoking in the LGBTQ+ population.

CDC website. Lesbian, Gay, Bisexual, and Transgender Persons and Tobacco Use. Accessed February 2022.

HEALTHCARE INSURANCE: TOO BIG TO BARGAIN WITH

Michael Flor's story.

The Seattle Times. Coronavirus survival comes with a $1.1 million, 181-page price tag. June 12, 2020.

Hurricane Andrew in 1992 bankrupted many home, vehicle, and business insurers as a result of payouts totaling $15.5 billion.

Insurance Information Institute. Hurricane Andrew and Insurance: The Enduring Impact of an Historic Storm. August 2012.

Medicare and Medicaid have nearly double the enrollees of the biggest private insurer, UnitedHealthcare Group.

Statista.com, Accessed February 2022.

The Department of Justice gave the go-ahead for a $69 billion merger between Aetna and CVS health.

CNBC. CVS creates new health-care giant as $69 billion merger with Aetna officially closes. November 28, 2018.

A subsidiary of United Health Group named Optum helped to fix the disastrous Obamacare website.

Newsweek. Thanks for Nothing: Obamacare Website Bunglers Fired. August 6, 2014.

Some insurance analysts are speculating healthcare insurers may need bailouts due to payouts for COVID-19 medical bills.

Zero Hedge. Coronavirus Medical Bills: America's Next Financial Crisis? February 12, 2021.

By 2026, it's estimated that $1 in every $5 spent in America will be spent on healthcare

Centers for Medicare and Medicaid Services, "NHE Fact Sheet." Accessed February 2022.

$200 is around the market rate for an hour of an ER doctor's time.

ACEP Now. 2019-2020 Emergency Physicians Compensation Report. October 2019.

People with better healthcare insurance can be charged more out-of-pocket than those without healthcare insurance.

The Wall Street Journal. How Much Does a C-Section Cost? At One Hospital, Anywhere from $6,241 to $60, 584. February 11, 2021.

AHA vs HHS lawsuit.

AHA and Plaintiffs v. Alex M. Azar II. Filed December 4, 2019.

By 2022, only about 14% of hospitals complied with the price transparency rule.

Becker's Hospital Review. 14% of hospitals compliant with price transparency survey finds: 4 things to know. February 10, 2022.

Some hospitals used search engine de-optimization tools and other tricks to hide price webpages were from Google and other search engines.

The Wall Street Journal. Hospitals Hide Pricing Data From Search Results. March 22, 2021.

CMS' Keystone ACO

CMS ACO Learning System Case Study. Keystone ACO's Health Navigator Program to Identify and Close Care Gaps. October 2019.

One-quarter of patients on government-run insurance plans are in an ACO, but the total annual cost savings to taxpayers was around $300 million out of trillions of dollars in expenditures in 2017.

Modern Healthcare. Medicare ACOs saved CMS $314 million in 2017. August 30, 2018.

Doctor convicted of Medicare fraud was involved in plans to build a water park in the Dominican Republic.

Department of Justice Press Release. Operator of Miami HIV Clinic Sentenced to 57 Months in Prison for Role in Medicare Fraud Ring. November 18, 2020

Doctors who are billing outliers for Medicare are known.

ProPublica. Medicare Billing Outliers Often Have Disciplinary Problems, Too. June 20, 2014.

Many patients undergoing ground and air ambulance transport receive out-of-network bills.

Most Patients Undergoing Ground and Air Ambulance Transportation Receive Sizable Out-Of-Network Bills. *Health Affairs.* Vol 39, No 5. April 2020.

A 2010 study found one-third of ER visits and one-quarter of hospital inpatient admissions triggered some type of out-of-network charge.

Sun EC, et al. Assessment of Out-of-Network Billing for Privately Insured Patients Receiving Care in In-Network Hospitals. *Journal of the American Medical Association Internal Medicine.* 2019;179(11):1543–1550.

Two-thirds of hospital ERs are staffed by independent contractor groups.

Cooper, et al. Surprise! Out-of-Network Billing for Emergency Care in the United States. *Journal of Political Economy*. Vol 128, No 9. September 2020.

A couple in New York was charged $257,000 out-of-pocket for obstetric and neonatology services after their prematurely born daughter died.

The New York Times. Their Baby Died in the Hospital. Then Came the $257,000 Bill. September 21, 2021.

THE CDC & NIH: PERPETUATING PROBLEMS TO PERPETUATE EXISTENCE

The CDC grew out of a 1946 merger between the US Public Health Service and the military's WWII Malaria Control in War Areas program (supported by the Rockefeller Foundation).

Parascandola J. From MCWA to CDC--origins of the Centers for Disease Control and Prevention. *Public Health Reports*. 1996;111(6):549-551.

DDT kills wildlife, contaminates crops, and can cause cancer in humans.

National Center for Biotechnology Information. PubChem Compound Summary. Retrieved February 2022.

Malaria was eradicated from the US around 1951.

The Imaginations of Unreasonable Men: Inspiration, Vision, and Purpose in the Quest to End Malaria. By Bill Shore. PublicAffairs. 2012.

In 1932, the US PHS began a study of untreated syphilis in African American males in the city of Tuskegee, Alabama.

Examining Tuskegee: The Infamous Syphilis Study and its Legacy. By Susan Reverby. Chapel Hill: The University of North Carolina Press. 2009.

The US PHS published a paper in 1934 detailing the ill effects of untreated syphilis on the body.

Mays VM. The Legacy of the U. S. Public Health Services Study of Untreated Syphilis in African American Men at Tuskegee on the Affordable Care Act and Health Care Reform Fifteen Years After President Clinton's Apology. *Ethics & Behavior*. 2012;22(6):411-418.

In 1943, three US Marine Hospital physicians discovered that penicillin completely cured syphilis when administered in the primary or secondary stage, but not after the infection progressed to latent or tertiary syphilis.

Furman, Bess. A Profile of the United States Public Health Service, 1798–1948. 1973. U.S. Department of Health, Education, and Welfare.

The CDC continued following men enrolled in the Tuskegee Experiment until a whistleblower came forward in 1972.

The Associated Press / The New York Times. "Syphilis Victims in U.S. Study Went Untreated for 40 Years". July 26, 1972.

Historians believe that due to the Tuskegee Experiment perhaps over a hundred men likely died of untreated syphilis, and at least 40 female partners contracted the disease, with at least 19 children being born with congenital syphilis.

Kim, Oliver J., Magner, Lois N. A History of Medicine. 2018. Taylor & Francis Group.

&

Final Report of the Tuskegee Syphilis Study Ad Hoc Advisory Panel. April 1973. For the U.S. Department of Health, Education, and Welfare, Public Health Service.

The National Foundation for Infantile Paralysis in the 1950s used donations to organize a polio vaccine clinical trial with 1.8 million pediatric participants.

Smithsonian Institute website. Whatever Happened to Polio? Accessed February 2022.

A bad batch of polio vaccine caused 250 cases of actual polio.

The Washington Post. The tainted polio vaccine that sickened and fatally paralyzed children in 1955. April 14, 2020.

Of the CDC's requested $6.6 billion budget in 2020, nearly half of that money went abroad ($2.6 billion to global efforts to fight tuberculosis, Ebola, and malaria, and $457 million to general "global disease protection programs").

CDC Budget Request Overview FY 2020.

Between 1984 and 1989, the CDC sent strains of anthrax bacteria, botulinum toxin, and West Nile virus to the University of Baghdad.

Associated Press. Iraq got seeds for bioweapons from U.S. October 1, 2002.

United Nations (UN) weapons inspector Jonathan Tucker commented on the CDC's shipments of biologic agents to Iraq, "...they [CDC] did deliver samples that Iraq said had a legitimate public health purpose, which I think was naïve to believe."

Associated Press. U.S. Supplied Germs to Iraq in '80s. October 1, 2002.

Post-9/11, the CDC's mission statement was updated to include national security language such as, "safety and security threats" and "health security."

CDC website. CDC Mission, Role, and Pledge. Accessed February 2022. Available at:

The CDC Foundation's Programs contain global projects that do not impact Americans.

CDC Foundation website. CDC Foundation Programs. Accessed February 2022.

The CDC Foundation's board members and advisors are a who's who list of insurance, hospital, academic, and think tank strategists.

CDC Foundation website. CDC Foundation Board Members. Accessed February 2022.

CDC statement: "Bartenders and servers in LGBT nightclubs are exposed to high levels of secondhand smoke."

CDC website. Lesbian, Gay, Bisexual, and Transgender Persons and Tobacco Use. Accessed February 2022.

Doctor advising people to wear four masks to prevent COVID-19 infection.

BGR.com. If you want the most COVID protection, one doctor says wearing 4 face masks is best. January 29, 2021.

CDC Director Dr. Brenda Fitzgerald resigned after it was revealed she bought shares in a tobacco company while CDC Director.

Politico. CDC director who traded tobacco stock resigns. January 31, 2018.

Polls that show that Americans' trust in the CDC is falling.

TheHill.com. Polls show trust in scientific political institutions eroding. September 15, 2020.

CDC proponents are rallying to try and turn that tide of souring public opinion.

Rasmussen SA, et al. Protecting the Editorial Independence of the CDC From Politics. *Journal of the American Medical Association*. 2020;324(17):1729–1730.

&

CNBC. Biden's incoming CDC director says Trump administration has 'muzzled' scientists: 'I have to fix that'. January 19, 2021.

From an initial budget of $4 million in 1947, Congress has exponentially grown the NIH's budget to nearly $42 billion in 2020.

NIH Budget Appropriations for FY 2020. Accessed February 2020.

NIH engaged in lax oversight of the EcoHealth Alliance's activities at the Wuhan Institute of Virology in China.

ZeroHedge. NIH Officials Allowed EcoHealth Alliance to Self-Police Risky Gain-of-function Experiments in Wuhan. November 4, 2021.

The NIH is the largest funder of biomedical research in the world.

Viergever, R.F., Hendriks, T.C.C. The 10 largest public and philanthropic funders of health research in the world: what they fund and how they distribute their funds. *Health Research Policy & Systems*. 2016.

EcoHealth Alliance applied for a Department of Defense grant with a proposal that included what grant reviewers considered risky gain-of-function research.

The Intercept. Leaked Grant Proposal Detail High-Risk Coronavirus Research. September 23, 2021. Available

Most NIH R01 grants go to older, white, men.

NIH Extramural Nexus Blog. Long-term trends in the age of principal investigators supported for the first time on NIH R01-Equivalent awards. November 18, 2021.

&

Ginther DK, et al. Race, ethnicity, and NIH research awards. *Science*. 2011;333(6045):1015-1019.

How universities get to spend indirect cost money from NIH grants.

NIH website. NIH Office of Management. Indirect Cost: Definition and Example. Accessed February 2022.

The stated aim of many MK-ULTRA projects was to help advance the treatment of addiction, depression, and other mental health problems.

Alliance for Human Research Protection. A vast web of clandestine collaborations between medical academics and the CIA. January 18, 2015.

Ted Kaczynski may have been an unwitting subject of an MK-ULTRA experiment.

The Atlantic. Harvard and the Making of the Unabomber. June 2000 Issue.

A $3 million NIH grant was for research that administered the psychiatric drug lithium to children younger than 10 years of age, an age range which was not authorized by the study's safety protocol.

ProPublica. The $3 Million Research Breakdown. April 26, 2018.

A study funded by NIH run by Columbia University is asking teenagers to divulge details of their sexual activity in exchange for hundreds of dollars of compensation.

ClinicalTrials.gov website. A Pragmatic Clinical Trial of MyPEEPS Mobile to Improve HIV Prevention Behaviors in Diverse Adolescent Men Who Have Sex with Men. Accessed February 2022.

A STAT investigation found that many researchers fail to report or fail to timely report study results to ClinicalTrials.gov.

STAT News. Failure to report: A STAT investigation of clinical trials reporting. December 13, 2015.

Many Fogarty grants are for research that does not affect Americans in the US.

The John Edward Fogarty International Center website. Americans benefit from global health research. Accessed February 2022.

&

NIH Fogarty International Center website. Fogarty Programs. Accessed February 2022.

In 2012 NIH announced that China, Russia, Turkey, and other Russia-friendly Baltic states were ineligible for Fogarty grants.

Notice of Change in Country Eligibility for Fogarty International Training Grants. Notice Number: NOT-TW-12-011. Release Date May 11, 2012.

The 2018 US Senate Committee on Homeland Security and Governmental Affairs report of China's Thousand Talents program detailed the NIH's unwitting role in the Chinese government's goals of stealing intellectual property from the United States.

United States Senate Permanent Subcommittee on Investigations, Committee on Homeland Security and Governmental Affairs. Threats to the U.S. Research Enterprise: China' Talent Recruitment Plans. Staff Report. 2018.

A Department of Justice investigation identified nearly 400 suspected participants in the Thousand Talents Program who had received NIH funding.

The Washington Times. More than 50 scientists fired or resign after NIH probe into grants' foreign support. June 17, 2020.

Anthony Fauci is, as of this writing, the highest paid federal government employee.

Forbes. Dr. Anthony Fauci: The Highest Paid Employee in the Entire U.S. Federal Government. January 25, 2021.

Responding to HIV in the 1980s and to the post-9/11 anthrax attacks, Fauci redirected NIAID's budget towards completely unsuccessful efforts to develop HIV and anthrax vaccines.

The Federalist. A short history of how Anthony Fauci has kept failing up since 1984. January 13, 2021.

The US military forced an anthrax vaccine on its soldiers and those who refused were discharged or harshly punished.

Military Times. Troops who refused anthrax vaccine paid a high price. June 17, 2021.

The NSF funded a $3 million grant studying how shrimp run on treadmills underwater.

The Chronicle of Higher Education. How a $47 shrimp treadmill became a $3-million political plaything. November 13, 2014.

PCORI was created by the Affordable Care Act, operates with annual budgets north of $2 billion, and is run by a board of directors that reports to no one.

PCORI website. In Brief PCORI Funding Reauthorization. 2020.

PCORI-funded projects include $6.8 million for "Leveraging mHealth and Peers to Engage African-Americans and Latinxs in HIV care," and $1.4 million for "Peer online motivational interviewing for sexual and gender minority male survivors."

PCORI 2019 Annual Report.

AHRQ's budget was $436 million in 2021.

Agency for Healthcare Research and Quality Operating plan for FY 2021.

The Pandemic Playbook

Heavy.com. How to read Obama's Pandemic Playbook PDF. May 15, 2020.

There are federal databases to track those who have not received a COVID-19 vaccination.

The Epoch Times. 25 Federal Agencies Tracking Employees with Religious Exemption Requests. January 19, 2022.

Initially many doctors believed the 1918 influenza pandemic was caused by a bacterium.

The Great Influenza: The Story of the Deadliest Plague in History. John M. Barry. Viking Press, New York, New York, 2004.

HIV was initially thought to be a cancer, and its mechanism of transmission was unknown for years.

CDC. *MMWR.* AIDS: the Early Years and CDC's Response. 2011;60(04):64-69.

Government healthcare agencies now spend $1 out of every $4 dollars in the federal budget.

The American Conservative. How to Fix Healthcare In America. October 21, 2020.

BIG PHARMA & THE FDA: REGULATORY CAPTURE

"The corpse to which we are chained."

Quote attributed to a WWI German Official regarding Germany's alliance with the Austro-Hungarian Empire.

Federal laws allow pharmaceutical companies to avoid liability for their products, specifically vaccines.

42 US Code 300aa-22.

About half of physicians receive payments from industry.

ProPublica. We Found Over 700 Doctors Who Were Paid More Than a Million Dollars by Drug and Medical Device Companies. October 17, 2019.

Payments from industry influence doctors' prescription patterns.

ProPublica. Doctors Prescribe More of a Drug If They Receive Money from a Pharma Company Tied to It. October 17, 2019.

A 2019 Gallup poll reported that three-quarters of Americans surveyed said the cost of prescription medicines would influence their presidential vote.

West Health & Gallup. The U.S. Healthcare Crisis. April 2019.

The average American spends around $1,229 each year on prescription and over-the-counter drugs.

Organization for Economic Co-operation and Development. Pharmaceutical Spending. Accessed February 2022.

The majority of Americans have less than $1,000 in savings.

Statista. Most Americans Lack Savings. December 18, 2019.

The reported median cost to develop a drug ranges from $648 million to $985 million, with a potential payoff of a median total revenue of $1.66 billion

Wouters OJ, et al. Estimated Research and Development Investment Needed to Bring a New Medicine to Market, 2009-2018. *Journal of the American Medical Association.* 2020;323(9):844–853.

&

Prasad V, Mailankody S. Research and Development Spending to Bring a Single Cancer Drug to Market and Revenues After Approval. *Journal of the American Medical Association Internal Medicine.* 2017;177(11):1569–1575.

In the age of machine learning, drug molecule development and testing are largely performed by supercomputers running algorithms and repeated simulations.

Rodriguez, S., et al. Machine learning identifies candidates for drug repurposing in Alzheimer's disease. *Nature Community.* 2021;12,1033.

Sometimes candidate drug molecules are tested using cells from aborted fetuses.

McKenna KC. Use of Aborted Fetal Tissue in Vaccines and Medical Research Obscures the Value of All Human Life. *Linacre Quarterly*. 2018;85(1):13-17.

The NIH spends over 50% of its budget searching for promising molecules and trying to better understand how diseases impair bodily function at the cellular level.

NIH website. NIH Office of Budget. Spending History by Institute, 1983 to present.

The FDA approved 210 new molecular entities between 2010-2016, and NIH studies either identified or contributed to work on every single one of those molecules.

Galkina Cleary E, et al. Contribution of NIH funding to new drug approvals 2010-2016. *PNAS.* 2018;115(10):2329-2334.

The original SARS vaccine trials did not end well for the monkeys, with antibody-dependent enhancement causing lung disease and death.

Tseng C-T, et al. Immunization with SARS Coronavirus Vaccines Leads to Pulmonary Immunopathology on Challenge with the SARS Virus. *PLOS ONE.* 2011;7(4): e35421.

Reference for the lengths of Phase 1-3 clinical trials.

Pregelj L, et al. Changes in clinical trial length. *Nature Reviews Drug Discovery*. 2015;14(5):307-8.

Over the last decade the NIH has itself performed more and more of those Phase 1-3 clinical trials on behalf of the pharmaceutical industry.

NIH News Releases. Five more pharmaceutical companies join NIH initiative to speed therapeutic discovery. June 12, 2012.

About 70% of drugs move on from Phase 1 to Phase 2, and about 30% of drugs move on from Phase 2 to Phase 3.

FDA website. Step 3: Clinical Research. Accessed February 2022.

Big pharma's in-house statisticians analyze the data from all Phases of clinical trials.

DrugWatch. Big Pharma's Role in Clinical Trials. April 24, 2015.

In "intent to treat analysis," statisticians can use data collected up until the time of the subject's exit from the study to favorably support the drug's efficacy,

McCoy CE. Understanding the Intention-to-treat Principle in Randomized Controlled Trials. *Western Journal of Emergency Medicine.* 2017;18(6):1075-1078.

"Pragmatic" statistical designs allow inclusion of data from people who forget to take their drug for days or even weeks, which may make a drug seem to have less frequent or fewer side effects.

Ford I, Norrie J. Pragmatic Trials. *New England Journal of Medicine.* 2016 Aug 4;375(5):454-63.

"Crossover" designs have participants who begin the trial taking the investigational drug eventually switch over to the placebo, and vice-versa.

Kane PB, et al. Individualized therapy trials: navigating patient care, research goals and ethics. *Nature Medicine.* 2021;27:1679-1686.

Remdesivir was studied for the treatment of COVID-19 using an adaptive clinical trial design.

NIH website. Accelerating COVID-19 Therapeutic Interventions and Vaccines (ACTIV). Accessed February 2022.

Between 2000-2011, 102 drug trials were retracted, 73 for scientific misconduct and 29 for statistical or other reporting errors.

Samp JC, et al. Retracted Publications in the Drug Literature. *Pharmacotherapy*. 2012;32(7):586-595.

Many principal investigators of trials and authors of clinical practice guidelines from academic universities are also receiving industry funding.

STAT News. Financial conflicts of interest in clinical practice guidelines remain an 'intractable problem.' October 29, 2018.

Only 25% of pharmaceutical companies are sharing any kind of data with the public.

Miller J, et al. Sharing of clinical trial data and results reporting practices among large pharmaceutical companies: cross sectional descriptive study and pilot of a tool to improve company practices. *British Medical Journal.* 2019;366:l4217.

Whistleblower report from the Pfizer's COVID-19 vaccine trials

Thacker P D. Covid-19: Researcher blows the whistle on data integrity issues in Pfizer's vaccine trial. *British Medical Journal.* 2021;375:n2635.

Hydroxychloroquine costs around $3.70 per pill.

Drugs.com. Accessed February 2022.

The study that initially convinced many doctors hydroxychloroquine was ineffective in treating COVID-19 and was dangerous to patients was retracted.

NBC News. The Lancet retracts large study on hydroxychloroquine. June 4, 2020.

Many physicians are concerned that use of Remdesivir increases mortality by causing organ failure.

Zampino, R., et al. Liver injury in remdesivir-treated COVID-19 patients. *Hepatology International.* 2020;14, 881–883.

The high efficacy rates initially reported in Phase 3 trials for the Western COVID-19 vaccines appear to approach zero well within a year's time.

Nordström, Peter et al. Effectiveness of Covid-19 Vaccination Against Risk of Symptomatic Infection, Hospitalization, and Death Up to 9 Months: A Swedish Total-Population Cohort Study. *The Lancet* pre-print. Posted October 25, 2021.

Eli Lilly & Co.'s Humalog, a type of fast-acting insulin, cost $21 a vial in 1996.

Hearing on "Priced Out of a Lifesaving Drug: The Human Impact of Rising Insulin Costs." Submitted to the United States House Committee on Energy & Commerce Oversight and Investigations Subcommittee. Testimony of Kasia J Lipska, MD, MHS. April 2, 2019.

After a decade of control by Mylan, the EpiPen package cost over $600, reaping annual sales of $1 billion for Mylan.

Seven Pillars Institute. Mylan's Epipen pricing scandal. September 14, 2017.

Mylan also gave money to pharmacy benefit managers in exchange for placing Mylan's EpiPens on pharmacies' preferred list of drugs that are recommend to customers.

Drug Delivery Business News. Mylan must face Epipen racketeering lawsuit. January 21, 2021.

Drug expiration dates are typically not accurate.

Propublica. The Myth of Drug Expiration Dates. July 18, 2017.

For many drugs, more important than the arbitrary expiration date is the temperature at which drugs are stored.

Patil Armenian, et al. Hot and Cold Drugs: National Park Service Medication Stability at the Extremes of Temperature. *Prehospital Emergency Care.* 2017;21:3:378-385.

Circa 2016, US citizens spent $480 billion on pharmaceutical drugs.

The IQVIA Institute. Medicines Use and Spending in the US. A Review of 2017 and Outlook to 2021. Institute Report, May 2017.

Pre COVID-19, Pfizer's annual gross profits were between $30 - 40 billion.

MacroTrends website. Pfizer Gross Profit 2006-2021. Accessed February 2022.

Pharmaceutical companies' profit margins are on par with Wall Street big banks.

DeAngelis CD. Big Pharma Profits and the Public Loses. *Milbank Quarterly*. 2016;94(1):30-33.

There are major drug shortages in the US currently.

Ventola CL. The drug shortage crisis in the United States: causes, impact, and management strategies. *Pharmacy and Therapeutics*. 2011;36(11):740-757.

NPR framed Donald Trump's interest in lowering drug prices as a "reckless attack" on hard-working companies.

NPR. Trump signs new executive order on prescription drug prices. September 13, 2020.

Purdue Pharma pled guilty to criminal charges, was fined $4.5 billion, and the company was dissolved.

The New York Times. Purdue Pharma is Dissolved and Sacklers Pay $4.5 Billion to Settle Opioid Claims. September 1, 2021.

New, ultra-potent opioids are still approved by the FDA.

NBC News. FDA approves powerful new opioid in 'terrible' decision. November 2, 2018.

&

FDA News Release. FDA approves new opioid for intravenous use in hospitals, other controlled clinical settings. August 7, 2020.

&

NPR. Despite warnings, FDA approves potent new opioid painkiller. November 2, 2018.

The FDA regulates over $1 trillion of products annually.

Smithsonian Magazine. Where did the FDA come from, and what does it do? February 8, 2017.

The FDA inspector assigned to thalidomide, Dr. Frances Kelsey, stalled the approval and asked for studies proving the drug did not affect developing fetuses.

The New York Times. Frances Oldham Kelsey, Who Saved U.S. Babies from Thalidomide, Dies at 101. August 8, 2015.

Prevalence of statin use amongst Americans

Salami JA, et al. National Trends in Statin Use and Expenditures in the US Adult Population From 2002 to 2013: Insights From the Medical Expenditure Panel Survey. *Journal of the American Medical Association Cardiology.* 2017;2(1):56–65.

A meta-analysis found that to prevent 18 people from having a stroke or a heart attack, 1,000 people each had to take a statin for 5 consecutive years.

Taylor F, et al. Statins for the primary prevention of cardiovascular disease. *Cochrane Database of Systematic Reviews.* 2013;1:CD004816.

Seven of the ten steps of the American College of Cardiology's Guideline on the Management of Blood Cholesterol advise initiating a statin or combinations of statins.

Grundy SM, Stone NJ. 2018 American Heart Association/American College of Cardiology Multisociety Guideline on the Management of Blood Cholesterol: Primary Prevention. *Journal of the American Medical Association Cardiology.* 2019;4(5):488-489.

Statins can cause rhabdomyolysis.

Mendes P, et al. Statin-induced rhabdomyolysis: a comprehensive review of case reports. *Physiotherapy Canada.* 2014;66(2):124-132.

Statins have been linked to weakening of the heart's muscle.

Silver MA, et al. Effect of atorvastatin on left ventricular diastolic function and ability of coenzyme Q10 to reverse that dysfunction. *American Journal of Cardiology.* 2004;94(10):1306-10.

Statins can increase the risk of developing Type II diabetes.

Mansi I, et al. Statins and New-Onset Diabetes Mellitus and Diabetic Complications: A Retrospective Cohort Study of US Healthy Adults. *Journal of General Internal Medicine.* 2015;30(11):1599-610.

&

Dormuth Colin R, et al. Higher potency statins and the risk of new diabetes: multicentre, observational study of administrative databases. *British Medical Journal.* 2014;348:g3244

The FDA describes the increased risk of developing Type II diabetes while on statins as a risk of "higher blood sugar."

FDA Drug Safety Communication: Important safety label changes to cholesterol-lowering statin drugs. Safety Announcement February 2012.

Statins also can cause liver failure and are linked to autoimmune diseases.

de Jong HJI, et al. Pattern of risks of rheumatoid arthritis among patients using statins: A cohort study with the clinical practice research datalink. *PLOS One.* 2018;13(2):e0193297.

Statin "calculators" essentially put anyone over the age of 65 on a statin regardless of their cholesterol levels.

Heart Risk Calculator based on ASCVD algorithm. Available at www.cvriskcalculator.com. Accessed February 2022.

Less than a year after facilitating the emergency use authorization for Moderna's COVID-19 vaccine, FDA commissioner Stephen Hahn became Chief Medical Officer at Flagship Pioneering, the venture capital firm that helped launch Moderna.

The Hill. Stephen Hahn joining venture capital firm behind Moderna. June 15, 2021.

The FDA's black box warning for ACE inhibitors advises against their use in pregnant women due to the risk of birth defects.

FDA website. Angiotensin-Converting Enzyme Inhibitor Drugs. Accessed February 2022.

The estimated incidence of angioedema from ACE inhibitors is 0.1-0.7%.

Vincenzo Montinaro, Marco Cicardi. ACE inhibitor-mediated angioedema, *International Immunopharmacology*. 2020;78:106081.

Bottle of Lies book about the FDA's attempted regulation of generic drugs made overseas and stateside.

Katherine Eban. *Bottle of Lies: The Inside Story of the Generic Drug Boom.* 2019. Harper Collins, New York, NY.

There have been issues with contaminated medicines from EpiPen manufacturer Mylan Pharmaceuticals and tainted doses of Johnson & Johnson COVID-19 vaccines made in Baltimore.

Biopharm Dive. FDA scolds Mylan for 'repeated' manufacturing problems. September 4, 2020.

&

The New York Times. A troubled vaccine plant in Baltimore is given the go ahead to reopen. July 29, 2021.

Thyroid medications have been recalled for not containing the actual active ingredient.

NBC News Washington. More thyroid drugs recalled because they may not be strong enough. September 21, 2020.

Examples of the FDA responding to issues with letters instead of concrete actions.

Politico. Whistleblower says FDA minimized safety risks at Merck vaccine plant. March 31, 2021.

&

Reuters. Special report: Insider alleges Eli Lilly blocked her efforts to sound alarms about U.S. drug safety. March 11, 2021.

From 2016-2019, the FDA switched to a shadow medical device reporting system called Alternative Summary Reporting.

Kaiser Health News. Hidden FDA Reports Detail Harm Caused by Scores of Medical Devices. March 7, 2019.

The CARES act's fines for unauthorized production of PPE were a $14,060 Monograph Drug Facility Fee and a $9,373 Contract Manufacturing Organization Facility Fee.

USA Today. HHS: Distilleries won't have to pay FDA fees of more than $14K for making hand sanitizers amid pandemic. December 31, 2020.

Researchers have explored NAC as a potential adjunct for the treatment of COVID-19.

Shi Z, Puyo CA. N-Acetylcysteine to Combat COVID-19: An Evidence Review. *Therapeutics and Clinical Risk Management.* 2020;16:1047-1055.

The FDA's letter to select NAC manufacturers stated that because NAC is FDA-approved for use as an antidote for acetaminophen overdose, that it cannot also be considered a dietary supplement.

Natural Products Insider. FDA warning letters on NAC cause stir in supplement sector. August 11, 2020.

VACCINES: IT DEPENDS WHAT THE MEANING OF 'IS' IS

The COVID vaccines are collectively the biggest blockbuster drug to date.

The New York Times. Pfizer's COVID vaccine could break record sales next year. November 2, 2021.

The CDC changed its definition of what vaccination means during the COVID-19 pandemic.

Sharyl Attkisson. CDC changes definition of "vaccines" to fit COVID-19 vaccine limitations. September 8, 2021.

Smallpox vials were reported to have been found at a laboratory in Pennsylvania.

NBC News Philadelphia. 'Smallpox' vials found at Merck lab in suburban Philadelphia Facility. November 17, 2021.

Influenza has been around since at least Hippocrates' time.

Barreto ML, et al. Infectious diseases epidemiology. *Journal of Epidemiology and Community Health.* 2006;60(3):192-195.

In the 1930s, backed by big pharma money, researchers (including Jonas Salk, future inventor of the polio vaccine) began trying to make a flu vaccine.

Francis T, Salk JE, Pearson HE, Brown PN. Protective effect of vaccination against induced Influenza A. *Journal of Clinical Investigation.* 1945;24(4):536-46.

The 1976 vaccine against the "Hong Kong" influenza caused hundreds of cases of paralysis in the United States.

BBC. The Fiasco of the US Swine Flu Affair of 1976. September 21, 2020.

Today's influenza vaccines do not prevent you from contracting the flu.

Keshavarz M, et al. Influenza vaccine: Where are we and where do we go? *Reviews in Medical Virology*. 2019;29(1):e2014.

Tamiflu is somewhat effective as an early therapeutic for the influenza virus.

Dobson J, et al. Oseltamivir treatment for influenza in adults: a meta-analysis of randomised controlled trials. *Lancet*. 2015;385(9979):1729-1737.

Monoclonal antibodies have been overall very effective for the early treatment of COVID-19.

Kreuzberger N, et al. SARS-CoV-2-neutralising monoclonal antibodies for treatment of COVID-19. *Cochrane Database Systemic Review.* 2021;9(9):CD013825.

The flu vaccine is a $6 billion annual business.

Fortune Business Insights. Influenza Vaccine Market Size, Share & COVID-19 Impact Analysis. Market Research Report July 2021.

Companies are thinking of designing flu vaccines with new mRNA technology.

CNBC. A universal flu vaccine may be the next big mRNA breakthrough for Moderna, Pfizer. January 10, 2022.

In response to COVID-19 vaccination, your cells collectively make trillions of spike proteins.

Stephanie Seneff and Greg Nigh. Worse than the disease? Reviewing some possible unintended consequences of the mRNA vaccines against COVID-19. *International Journal of Vaccine Theory, Practice, and Research.* 2021;2(1):38-79.

As of this writing, Novavax is trying to get approval in the US for a protein-based COVID vaccine.

Yahoo News. Novavax CEO explains delay in COVID-19 vaccine EUA filing. August 6, 2021.

French company Valneva failed to obtain UK government approval for an inactivated virus vaccine against COVID.

Reuters. UK PM Johnson disappointed Valneva COVID-19 shot did not gain approval. November 24, 2021.

The Moderna COVID vaccine is being blamed for some vaccine-induced injuries.

NPR. The FDA is proving whether the Moderna vaccine can cause a rare side effect in teens. October 31, 2021.

Worldwide, 29 companies were furiously working on developing COVID-19 vaccines as early as February 2020.

Mother Jones. Operation Warp Speed: A Timeline. November 23, 2020.

Pfizer, Johnson & Johnson, and Moderna Operation Warp Speed government contracts.

Congressional Research Service. Operation Warp Speed Contracts for COVID-19 Vaccines and Ancillary Vaccination Materials. Updated March 1, 2021. Accessed February 2022.

Some of those who have not taken a COVID-19 vaccination are highly educated individuals.

King WC, et al. Time trends, factors associated with, and reasons for COVID-19 vaccine hesitancy: A massive online survey of US adults from January-May 2021. *PLOS ONE.* 2021;16(12):e0260731.

Federal statute protects pharmaceutical companies from liability: "No vaccine manufacturer shall be liable in a civil action for damages arising from a vaccine-related injury or death associated with the administration of a vaccine."

42 US Code 300aa-22.

Individual physicians were granted immunity from liability related to administering COVID-19 vaccines by a March 2020 declaration from the Secretary of Health and Human Services, coinciding with the launch of Operation Warp Speed.

2020 Public Readiness and Emergency Preparedness (PREP) Act Declaration by Health and Human Services.

CONCLUSION

70% of patients treated in ERs do not have an actual emergency.

Truven Health Analytics Research Brief. 2013. Avoidable Emergency Department Usage Analysis.

Obesity dramatically increases the risk of dying from COVID-19.

Tartof SY, et al. Obesity and Mortality Among Patients Diagnosed With COVID-19: Results From an Integrated Health Care Organization. *Annals of Internal Medicine.* 2020;173(10):773-781.

Until the 1960s, medical malpractice litigation was extremely uncommon in the US.

Physician's News Digest. A Brief History of Medical Malpractice. May 10, 2017.

The average primary care appointment allots 15 minutes to discuss 6 topics.

Tai-Seale M, et al. Time allocation in primary care office visits. *Health Services Research.* 2007;42(5):1871-1894.

Doctors wait 11 seconds on average before interrupting a patient.

Forbes. How Long Can You Talk before Your Doctor Interrupts You. July 22, 2018.

Before the COVID-19 pandemic, medical errors were the third-leading cause of death in the US.

Makary MA, Daniel M. Medical error-the third leading cause of death in the US. *British Medical Journal.* 2016;353:i2139.

List of potential adverse effects from Pfizer COVID-19 vaccination

The South African. Pfizer's COVID vaccine has 1,291 rare side effects, own report shows. March 8, 2022.

CPSIA information can be obtained
at www.ICGtesting.com
Printed in the USA
LVHW100304300422
717322LV00005B/59